SPIRITUAL

BY

W. F. COBB, D.D.

RECTOR OF ST. ETHELBURGA'S IN THE CITY OF LONDON

AUTHOR OF "ORIGINES JUDAICÆ," "THEOLOGY OLD AND NEW."
"THE PSALMS," "MYSTICISM AND THE CREED," ETC.

- Bishop Berkeley
- Plato
idealistic philosophy
of non-matter.
"Spirit is the Sole form of reality."

1914

TO

IVO GEIKIE COBB, M.D.

THIS BOOK IS DEDICATED BY THE AUTHOR

IN TOKEN OF LOVE AND

RESPECT

.

PREFACE

THE question of Spiritual Healing is one which has reappeared in an acute form during the past twenty years, and been the subject of much discussion and of great perplexity. Though little agreement has been reached about the *modus operandi* of Spiritual Healing in general, or of the nature of Faith, and though apparently even men of eminence have not thought out what they mean by "suggestion," yet no doubt now remains that we are face to face with a mode of curing disease other than that which orthodox medicine had hitherto recognized as valid. The difficulty of appraising this intruder on the sacred domain held in trust by the British Medical Council lies in the greater difficulty which we find lying across the path of all Science, viz. that of expressing Life in terms of Thought and of applying it to our daily needs as our willing servant. Life as the indeterminate factor of experience is reluctant to be locked up in forms and limited by tradition. And the slowness of the acceptance by medicine of hypnotism is a case in point.

The statement of Spiritual Healing, its history and nature, as given here, is meant to be popular, not technical; general, though (it is hoped) not superficial. The author's object has been to set out partly the facts which show that Spiritual Healing in some sense is more than a hallucination or a fraud, or a recrudescence of obsolete modes of thought; and partly to set forth the metaphysic which lies (as he thinks) embedded in the phenomena of Spiritual Healing. He feels that he has expressed very imperfectly the profound respect he feels for the achievements and the human spirit which adorn the medical profession, and it is this very respect which impels him to express a hope that, after having gone so far as to admit the claims of suggestion and hypnotism, they will go further, and add to the very proper caution which characterizes them, an open eye for the indications of healing powers which are at home in the supersensible world.

CONTENTS

CONTENTS

CHAPTER VII

CHAPTER VIII

CHAPTER IX

CHAPTER X

CHAPTER XI

CHAPTER XII

CHAPTER XIII

SPIRITUAL HEALING

INTRODUCTION

SPIRITUAL HEALING in some form or other meets us in all ages of which the history has been written. Though unknown by this distinctive title, it none the less occupies a large place in savage societies, and is found at later and more advanced stages of growth; and though the area of its activities may have been encroached on, it yet holds its own on its undisputed ground. Even in these days of modern scepticism it has taken on a fresh lease of life, and the activity and growth of Christian Science alone is sufficient to show that there is a vital tenacity about Spiritual Healing which defies the assaults and even the indifference of widely differing ages. The cause of that tenacity, and the place which Spiritual Healing occupies in promoting, or it may be in hindering, the well-being of man, it is the purpose of the following pages to set out.

There are, as usual, two courses open to an inquiry of this sort. We may start with a definition of what Spiritual Healing is, and then proceed to marshal the evidence in support of our *a priori* definition, or we may sketch at the beginning the facts we

B

have to account for, and then proceed to inquire
what theory or hypothesis will best classify and
explain them. It seems to us that the second course
is preferable, and for these reasons.

In the first place, it may be that the definition
selected may be true so far as it goes, and may be
well supported by the evidence, and yet may give
but a partial, and so far, therefore, an untrue
picture of the whole which the definition professes
to cover. I may, for example, start a discussion on
anthropology by defining man as a two-legged
animal without feathers, or as an animal which
prays, or an animal which uses fire, or one which
uses tools, and then prove my thesis triumphantly
by the evidence I choose to put in, while the evidence I have suppressed as irrelevant to my purpose
may be just the evidence which shows man to
embrace characteristics widely different from those
suggested by my definition. Similarly I may, if I
choose, define Spiritual Healing as the product of
subjective faith, of transmitted energy, of cosmic
force rightly applied, of religious zeal, as due to
right thinking, to subconscious forces, or to the
miraculous intervention of Deity, and then prove
by skilfully selected cases from history the right-
ness of the definition. And when this had been
done it should not be difficult for another to show
by the same method that another definition was
equally valid, and a third person to do the same
with a third definition, and so on.

A further advantage in the second method suggested is that it enables the author and his reader
to travel along the road pleasantly as companions

conversing on equal terms, each as well fitted as the other to judge on the evidence for the thesis about which they are discoursing. The first method would substitute for this free and equal relationship of fellow-travellers, the less human and perhaps less useful relation of guide and follower. And the follower would have no certainty before he reached his journey's end as to the trustworthiness of his guide. In any case, he deprives himself (or is deprived by his guide) of the joy which comes from adventuring along an unknown road without any guarantee against surprises.

In the third place, our second method has the inestimable advantage of forming, as it is put into action, a coherent, though more or less "subconscious," hypothesis about the facts as they pass across the stage. Then, when the author formulates his own hypothesis to account for the facts, the reader will bring forward his own half-formed solution in corroboration or contradiction. In this way he will in either case gain a more vivid sense of what the truth that is being sought is really like.

We shall begin, therefore, with a sketch of the facts which may serve to illustrate the nature of Spiritual Healing, premising only that the facts are never very sharply defined, and are apt, moreover, to become more and more difficult to seize as culture develops in new and strange directions. Thus our evidence might be expected to be most luxuriant in the early stages of culture, and to be scanty and difficult to drag into the cold light of criticism in more cultured times. On the other hand, the inequality between the two periods may be lessened by the greater quantity of records in the later as compared with the earlier.

Against all premature formulating of hypotheses there stands the powerful prejudice against Spiritual Healing entertained by the medical profession in general, and more particularly by many of its leading representatives. Nobody, it is fair to say, can be surprised at the obstinacy of this prejudice who reflects on the necessary conservatism of bodies of trustees on the one hand, and, on the other hand, considers the provocation frequently given by advocates of Spiritual Healing. Moreover, the medical profession, through its official representative, the British Medical Council (founded in 1858), is as imperfectly representative as the corresponding authority in the Established Church and in the Law, and it differs from these two latter in the important respect that no appeal lies from its decisions. Hence medical men are unduly handicapped in any attempt to give practical expression to progress in knowledge where it goes beyond established rules, and in all probability they are as a body less rigidly opposed to all change than their Council is. Yet it must be borne in mind that the medical profession is a trustee for the public, and is bound, therefore, to try all proposals for the adoption of new principles, though it does not seem bound, even if it were possible, to test officially new methods which fall within accepted principles. In the discharge of this trust, however, it cannot be said that the British Medical Council has shown more stiffness than the Church or the Law has shown in a similar position, even though in some recent cases its decisions may have seemed to many unduly harsh. And clearly it is not to be expected that medical authority should accept without much careful inquiry a proposal which, though old enough in itself, is to it officially new.

What medical science has a right to demand, and what the advocates of Spiritual Healing have not as a rule conceded, is, first, a rational ground for non-medical treatment, and, secondly, adequate evidence for alleged cures. It is not enough to lay stress on the ability of Life to cure disorders by its own inherent vigour, unless at the same time some effort, at all events, be made to chart the road along which this Life may be expected to travel on its journey of beneficence. And also the sensibilities of the mind trained in scientific habit are justly outraged when large claims are made and no evidence offered to show that an exact diagnosis has been made, and every precaution taken to exclude error, as well as to make it certain that a cure has been effected.

In the state of feeling, then, which has been brought into existence by the reluctance to abandon the old paths on the one hand, and by confident and ill-supported claims on the other, it would seem better that an inquiry into Spiritual Healing should go softly, and abstain from doing more than suggest a conclusion until the historical evidence has been adequately set out.

We shall have occasion later to discuss the psychological and metaphysical problems involved in the claim for the validity of Spiritual Healing. And it will be found that the battles of the schools appear even when we are trying to ascertain the nature and limits of the power of the spirit to heal the body. The ancient belief in demons raises the question of the nature of the Soul, and with the Soul is bound up the general relation of spirit and body. Even Zeno's puzzle about the immobility of the moving arrow and about Achilles and the tortoise reappears when we try to give an account of suggestion and its influence on the patient.[1] Our theory of Spiritual Healing if we think of God as merely transcending His world, will be different from our theory if we fix our eyes on His immanence only. So, too, if we hold the doctrine of a transcendental Self, we shall think differently from the way we should think if we contented ourselves with an empirical Ego. And if we take the sensualistic view of Matter we shall find difficulties in accepting Spiritual Healing as a fact which we shall not find if we treat it as mere negativity.

These philosophical difficulties are not those, however, with which the medical profession is concerned. Its difficulties are partly of a practical nature and partly scientific. It cannot under the former head commit itself to proposals which may needlessly endanger life or health, and under the latter it feels itself as a public trustee bound to scrutinize very carefully all new and unfamiliar claimants to scientific recognition. The general attitude of the profession may be gathered from the Report of the British Medical Council's Sub-Committee printed in Appendix A, from the Report of the mixed committee of doctors and clergy printed

[1] See Bergson, *Creative Evolution*, pp. 325–30.

in Appendix B, and from the official declarations of the *British Medical Journal*. For example, this journal writes [1] that it understands by faith-healing "the cure of disease without the intervention of any known physical agency"; that miracles "are not peculiar to any religion, Christian or other, and have been wrought by 'animal magnetizers' and healers of various kinds, who are not in any way associated with theological or spiritual formulas." It proceeds to say that "we have constantly maintained two propositions: (1) That it is foolish to declare dogmatically with Matthew Arnold, following Renan, that 'miracles' in this sense do not happen; (2) that the operative factor in Spiritual Healing is the ill-defined force known as 'suggestion.' It is, in very truth, the patient's faith that makes him whole. That faith can be excited by certain beliefs, by certain personalities, and very largely by 'imitation,' the potency of which was clearly recognized by the French Commission which reported on Mesmerism in 1784. Belief in 'miraculous' cures is like panic or enthusiasm—whether religious, military or political—in the highest degree contagious, and it is amid crowds of devout believers thronging around a famous shrine, with all the accessories that contribute to quicken faith into the force that 'moves mountains' that such events are most common." The journal then points out that there are limits to the curative power of faith which roughly correspond to the "boundary between diseases which are called 'functional' and those which are 'organic.'"

[1] December 16, 1911, p. 1609.

Now this attitude is, on the whole, wise and, within limits, well grounded. If we might substitute the indefinite for the definite article in the proposition that "*the* operative factor in Spiritual Healing is suggestion," and say that *an* operative factor is suggestion, we should then be saying what is incontrovertible. But in view of some of the cures, for example, worked at Lourdes it is hazardous to affirm that "suggestion," however far you extend its range, is the sole instrument of cure. And as we shall see in Chapter IX, the term "suggestion" is itself not much more than a label we find it convenient to use for a process which is still carried on in darkness for the greater part.

We might also demur to the definition assigned to the term "miracles," which limits them to the group of cures which are represented by those of "animal-magnetizers," for this (as we shall see in Chapter XII) omits that "supernatural" factor which is of the essence of any legitimate sense attributed to the term miracle.

Further, we might also, for the sake of clearness, point out [1] that the distinction between "functional" and "organic" is not only untenable scientifically, being only a term of convenience, a sort of rule of thumb, but also that "functional" itself labours under a serious ambiguity. It may mean that the phenomena it covers are thereby assigned to the realm of pure psychical causality, or it may also be used, and is frequently so used, as a convenient term for some unknown cause for which no "organic" correlate can be discovered. Thus a man suffering

[1] See below, p. 146 f.

from aphasia may baffle all attempts to discover an organic cause for his malady, and hence the practitioner will have no option but to diagnose it as "functional"—that is, as unknown. Just as Sir Francis Galton could write:[1] "The march of science is fast obliterating the distinction between the material and the non-material, for it is now generally admitted that matter is a microcosm of innumerable and it may be immaterial motes, and that the apparent vacancy of space is a plenum of ether that vibrates throughout like a solid," so we shall before long have to write that the march of physiological science is fast obliterating the distinction between the "functional" and the "organic."

That belief in Spiritual Healing may be easily exploited for purposes of gain is known to everybody, though it is not everybody who realizes how frequently it is done. One example of it may be given to put the unwary on their guard. Mr. John Adams Thayer published in 1911 a book[2] describing a campaign he undertook on behalf of what he called "clean advertising." Among his warning examples he cited the case of a Spiritual Healer, Francis Truth. "It is the press," he said, "of New England which should bear the odium of Francis Truth's shameless success. This quack, schooled to unusual cunning among fakers of the most dangerous type, easily found complaisant publishers to print his advertisements, headlines and all, in the guise of news. Thanks to their trumpeting of

---

[1] *The Times*, May 31, 1910.
[2] *Getting On: the Confessions of a Publisher.*

his miraculous 'cures,' he established himself luxuriously in one of Boston's best sections and surrounded himself with scores of clerks, who with series of manifolded letters 'treated' the stricken and deluded thousands who could not flock directly to his door. To those who did come he showed a trophy-room decorated with discarded canes, crutches and braces. Among these convincing relics were also displayed the charred ends of many expensive cigars, for even the smoking habit came within the range of his divine activities. When the crash came the office-boy testified that these stumps had been smoked by the healer himself, after his exhausting labours for ailing humanity. But there were profits before the crash, ten months of profits, which accumulated at the astounding figure of thirty thousand dollars (£6,000) a week. Then Francis Truth was placed under arrest. The publishers escaped." [1]

[1] See *British Medical Journal*, July 8, 1911, p. 84.

CHAPTER I

ONE feature in savage culture is common and striking. Medicine is the prerogative of the priesthood. And though we have no warrant for holding any savages described by missionaries, traders, or travellers to be "primitive," since behind them all is a long past, yet there is no reason for refusing to project backwards this alliance between healing and priestly functions. Moreover, whether we go to Mexico or Greece, Egypt or North America, we find that divination, or prophecy, goes hand in hand with healing, and that the god who presides over both is, as a rule, a chthonian deity. Healing as well as prophecy came from the gods, and the shaman, conjurer, sorcerer, medicine-man or wizard was the agent of the god, his priest and mouthpiece. Hence, as Dr. Brinton tells us,[1] their names among the Algonkins and Dakotas were : "those knowing divine things," "dreamers of the gods," "masters or guardians of the divine things," "those possessed of the divine fire," "the wise ones," and so forth. Sickness, like death, was regarded by the savage as abnormal, and therefore as due to supernatural agency, to the anger of a god, or to the use of a

[1] *Myths of the New World*, 1868, p. 264.

god's power by some powerful medicine-man. Hence the nature of the remedy was determined by the source of the disease, and Spiritual Healing took the form of enlisting the help of a god or spirit through a more powerful medicine-man, and with the ritual consecrated by usage and tradition.

The Cherokees have a belief (borrowed, it is possible, from Europe) that "the seventh son is a natural born prophet with the gift of healing by touch." [1]

Among the red men were medicine-women as well as medicine-men.

If Novalis is right when he says that "prayer is in religion what thought is in philosophy; the religious sense prays as the reason thinks," then the Nootka Indian prayer given by Dr. Brinton tells us that the healing asked for in it must be assigned to a spiritual force : "Great Quahootze," it runs, "let me live, not be sick, find the enemy, not fear him, find him asleep and kill a great many of him." [2] This may be easily paralleled from the Psalms of David, e. g. "Remove thy stroke away from me." The whole of Psalm xxxviii. is a prayer that Jahweh would take away the leprosy from which the writer was suffering, and in Psalm cii. is the prayer, "O my God, take me not away in the midst of my days." The same sort of petition meets us in ancient Babylonia, with the difference that at that time the worshipper had not the same certainty

---

[1] Dr. MacGowan, *Amer. Hist. Mag.*, x. p. 139 ; Whipple, *Report on the Indian Tribes*, p. 35 ; Brinton, *ubi supra*, p. 322 ; Brinton, *Ibid.*, p. 281.

[2] Brinton, *Ibid.*, 1868, p. 297.

about the god to whom his appeal should be directed as the Jew afterwards attained.

Nor need we be deterred from appealing to the incantations used in Babylonia, for, as Sayce says, following Lenormant, "they go back to the age of animism, to the days when as yet the multitudinous spirits and demons of Sumerian belief had not made way for the gods of Semitic Babylonia, or the sorcerer and medicine-man for a hierarchy of priests. Their language, as well as their spirit, is Sumerian, and the Zi, or 'spirit' of heaven and earth, is invoked to repel the attack of the evil ghost, or to shower blessings on the head of the worshipper." [1] So "the pure waters which heal the sick and destroy the power of witchcraft are brought by the water-spirit Ninakha-Kudda, "the mistress of spells,' whom the theologians of a later time transformed into a daughter of Ea." [2] In the same way the medicine-man among the Indians "muttered a formula over a gourd filled from a neighbouring spring and sprinkled it (the water) on his patient, or washed the diseased part, or sucked out the evil spirit and blew it into a bowl of water, and then scattered the liquid on the fire or earth." [3]   That

[1] A. H. Sayce, *The Religions of Ancient Egypt and Babylonia*, 1902, p. 400.

[2] *Ibid.*, p. 407. *Cf.* "the hymns to the sun-god were not yet emancipated from the magical beliefs and ceremonies in which they had had their origin ; they were still incantations rather than hymns in the modern sense of the word. The collection to which they belonged must have been used by the class of priests known as 'Chanters,' or 'Enchanters,' who had succeeded to the sorceries of medicine-men of the pre-Semitic past." *Ibid.*, p. 415.

[3] Brinton, *ubi supra*, p. 147.

this is a case of Spiritual Healing is clear from the necessity of having a medicine-man, and this necessity in its turn witnesses to the nature of the cure as consisting in the expulsion of the disturbing spirit by spiritual means. We shall meet with the same underlying conceptions presently in Christian lustrations.

Incantations, indeed, in earlier culture do but set in motion the belief in magic which is general, and this belief in turn rests on the fallacies (as we hold them to be) that "antecedence and consequence in time are the same as cause and effect"; that "like affects like," and in general that "casual connection in thought is equivalent to causative connection in fact." Hence disease was magically caused, and could be magically removed. Nature, it was thought, was peopled by invisible spirits, and over these spirits magicians and sorcerers had influence. Thus we can easily understand the bearing on the history of Spiritual Healing of the following formula, dated 1700 B.C., from a medical papyrus in the Leipzig collection—

"May Isis deliver, deliver; Horus was delivered by Isis from all ill that was inflicted on him by his brother Set when he slew his father, Osiris. O Isis, mistress of sorceries, deliver me, set me free from all bad, evil, red things, from the power of illness coming from god, or goddess, from death male and female, from plague male and female that taketh hold upon me, even as thou didst set free thy son Horus." [1]

[1] A. Wiedemann, *Religion of the Ancient Egyptians*, 1897, p. 272 f.

What Wiedemann says of Egyptian magic may be safely taken as representative of magic in general, both on its evil side as an instrument of spiritual power for the undoing of its victim, and on its good side as an instrument of Spiritual Healing. "Magic could not only cause very disagreeable inconvenience, but it might also bring about death; there is a set of directions for visiting your enemy with shivering and fever—probably ague—until he is undone; in another place we are told how a man may be made to die of insomnia, and there is much more of the same kind. Absurd as the pretensions of the magicians may seem, the multitude thoroughly believed in them, and great was the fear of sorcerers and of sorcery. In Egypt magical doctrines were not mere popular superstitions; they were part of the religion of the land, which was largely based on magic, and always intimately connected with it." [1]

How persistent is this belief in magic is shown by its survival in days when Nature has been rationalized and her activities classified and brought under the concept of uniformity. Prayers are daily offered throughout the Christian world for the recovery of sick people. The weather not infrequently forms also the content of prayer, while success in war, trade or love is thought of as depending on our ability to affect in some way the will of the God to whom we pray. Lourdes, Christian Science, Bethshan are names which testify to a belief in the alteration of the natural by the supernatural (to use

---

[1] Wiedemann, *Religion of the Ancient Egyptians*, 1897, p. 282 f.

popular language) by means of our own efforts or God's grace. Whether this belief is a superstitious survival, or rests on a rational foundation, we shall have to inquire later on. But we cannot escape from one all-pervading belief which obtains through all more childlike faiths, has fallen into the background in these more rationalistic or mathematical days, but seems too deeply rooted in the nature of things to be excluded permanently—I mean, the belief in spirits.

But one point must be emphasized. Primitive healing rests on the presupposition of animism, the historical importance of which can hardly be exaggerated. "Spiritual philosophy has influenced every province of human thought, and the history of animism once clearly traced would record the development, not of religion only, but of philosophy, science and literature." According to Prof. E. B. Tylor, "the theory of *Animism* divides into two great dogmas, forming parts of one consistent doctrine; first, concerning souls of individual creatures, capable of continued existence after the death or destruction of the body; second, concerning other spirits, upward to the rank of powerful deities." [1] It is the second division which we are here concerned with, although, indeed, it is but a corollary to the first. According to it "the whole of the inanimate kingdom, as well as all animated beings, are endowed with reason, intelligence and volition, identical with that of man." [2] The phenomena which led to animism are such as trance and the exalted consciousness of intoxication of all kinds,

[1] *Primitive Culture*, i. 385.   [2] *Encyc. Brit.*, xi. ed., ii. 25.

clairvoyance, death, dreams, apparitions, hallucinations, shadows and swoons. And at the bottom of them all lies the inexpugnable necessity for beings like men of interpreting experience anthropomorphically, the difference between savage and cultured peoples in this respect being that the latter uses a large anthropomorphism and the former a smaller. To both, therefore, idealism in some sense is inevitable. But to the primitive mind it never seems to occur that change can be due to anything but spirit, or, rather, if that be thought too advanced a conception, to spirits. And these spirits are innumerable, and are not confined to the visible order.

Thus, Dr. Tylor tells us that among the Watchandis of Australia a man slain by another passes into the victor's body as a "woorie," or warning spirit; that in Tasmania a native will attribute his deliverance from an accident to his deceased father's spirit as his guardian angel; that among the North American Indians it is an important act of religion for the individual to secure his patron genius; that sorcerers among the Esquimaux practise their art by means of a familiar spirit which may be the soul of a deceased parent; that alike in Chili, among the Caribs, or the African negroes, and the Asiatic Mongols the same belief holds good.[1]

Grimm tells us [2] that the "wild-woman" who healed the far-famed Wate was a wise-woman, a half-goddess. He also refers to the Gudrunlied verses : "Hyfjaberg this rock is called, and has long

---

[1] *Primitive Culture,* 1891, p. 200 ff.
[2] *Teutonic Mythology,* Stallybrass, iii. 1148.

C

been to the sick and to wounds a solace; whole becomes any woman, though she have a year's sickness, if she climbs it." He adds that in ancient Germany prophetesses, Parcæ, Muses all are imagined dwelling on mountains, so that to the art of healing we have a right worshipful origin assigned. It is notable that in Old Norse *læknir* was a physician, and in Middle High German *lâchenære* a sorcerer (*cf.* our leech). This connection of terms helps us to understand how the medicine practised by Christian priests in the Middle Ages, with the saints and holy martyrs helping them, found its rival in the remedies prescribed by the wise women, and partly accounts for the persecution to which the ecclesiastical authorities subjected the witches. They were rival Spiritual Healers.

Ancient belief was largely animistic, and it was not in Palestine alone that sicknesses were regarded as imposed by demons. Homer says "the demon afflicts, the compassionate god heals." Diseases were even personified, so that in the Edda "an oath is exacted from *diseases* as from living creatures to do no harm to Balder."

Grimm also quotes an ancient spell in narrative form : [1] "Nesia the harmful was wandering along different roads seeking whom she might injure; the Lord met her, and said : 'Nesia, whither goest thou?' 'I am going to the servant of God, N., to irritate his bones, soften his nerves, dry up his flesh.' The Lord said to her : 'I charge thee in the

---

[1] *Teutonic Mythology,* iv. 1695.

name of the Father, etc., that thou leave the servant
of God and go into a desert place.' "

An instructive account of the method of curing
a patient among the Malays known as the ceremony
of invoking the Tiger Spirit is given by Mr. Skeat.
In the autumn of 1896 he was enabled to be present
at the ceremony with others, the number in all
being always uneven, and the ceremony being
gone through as a rule on three consecutive nights.
The medicine-man, after fumigating himself with
incense, lay down on his back and covered his face,
while an old woman was chanting a long invocation. Then "for some time we sat in the silence of
expectation. At length, however, the moment of
possession arrived, and with a violent convulsive
movement which was startling in its suddenness,[1]
the 'Pawang' rolled over on to his face. Again
a brief interval ensued, and a second but somewhat
less violent spasm shook his frame, the spasm being
strangely followed by a dry and ghostly cough. A
moment later and the Pawang, still with shrouded
head, was seated bolt upright facing the tambourine
player."

Next there followed a number of ceremonies,
which found their climax in the stroking of the
patient with a sheaf of palm-blossom. After which
the Pawang sank back exhausted on the floor.

"A long interval now ensued, but at length,
after many convulsive twitchings, the shrouded
figure arose, amid the intense excitement of the

---

[1] Those who have been present at spiritualistic séances will
recall the similar convulsive movements which mark the beginning of the medium's trance-state.

entire company, and went upon its hands and feet. The Tiger Spirit had taken possession of the Pawang's body, and presently a low but startingly lifelike growl—the unmistakable growl of the dreaded ' Lord of the Forest ' seemed to issue from somewhere under our feet as the weird, shrouded figure began scratching furiously at the mat upon which it had been quietly lying, and then, with occasional pauses for the emission of the growls which had previously startled us, and the performance of wonderful catlike leaps, rapidly licked up the handfuls of rice which had been thrown upon the floor in front of it. This part of the performance lasted, however, but a few minutes, and then the evident excitement of the onlookers was raised to fever pitch as the bizarre and, as it seemed to our fascinated senses, strangely brute-like form stooped suddenly forward and slowly licked over, as a tigress would lick its cub, the all but naked body of the patient. . . . Reverting to a sitting posture the Pawang now leaned forward over the patient, and with the point of his dagger drew blood from his own arm ; then rising to his feet he engaged in a fierce hand-to-hand combat with his invisible foe (the spirit whom he had been summoned to exorcise). At first his weapon was the dagger, but before long he discarded this, and laid about him stoutly enough with the sheaf of areca-palm blossom." [1]

Mr. Skeat does not say whether the patient recovered. He quotes, however, from Swetten-

---

[1] W. W. Skeat, *Malay Magic*, 1900, p. 436 ff.

ham [1] a description of a similar ceremony in which
a very superior Spirit was invoked, one of four
Exalted Spirits, the guardians of the Sultan and
the State. In the ceremony the central figure was
the Sultan himself, seated on a sixteen-sided stand,
who was from time to time seized with a convulsive
shudder. Later the Sultan was found in a swoon,
during which the State Spirit, the first of the four
Exalted Spirits, was supposed to take possession
of the sick man's body. Here the king recovered,
and afterwards told the author that he "was not
himself and did not know what he was doing."

Advocates of the suggestion hypothesis will no
doubt account for phenomena of this sort by saying
that native belief was so strong that it set going
the necessary train of unquestioning expectations
which actualized themselves in the metamorphosis
of the Pawang. And they can appeal, no doubt, to
the phenomena of the *idée fixe* in hysteria and the
hallucinations to which it may give rise. But one
significant feature would still remain unaccounted
for, viz. the convulsive shuddering movement which
marks the entry on the alienation of consciousness.
This same feature reappears in the case of De
Rudder to be described afterwards when we come
to the "miracles" of Lourdes. The unconsciousness
of the Sultan to his surroundings reappears in the
case of Noémi Nightingale,[2] while the Lourdes
patients testify repeatedly to a feeling of returning
vigour coursing through their veins as accompanying their cure. Taking all these incidents together,

[1] *Malay Sketches*, pp. 153-9.   [2] See p. 112 below.

we shall hesitate before we conclude that "suggestion" alone can account for the results. We need not doubt that "suggestion" is a factor which may enter into the complex of forces working towards health, but even so we do not seem justified in assigning to it in many cases more than a subordinate rôle, and, further, we have not even then, by labelling this minor force "suggestion," done anything to explain its nature. This point will be discussed later on in Chapter IX.

CHAPTER II

SPIRITUAL HEALING IN THE GREEK WORLD

LET us now turn to the most famous healing cult of antiquity, that known in the worship of Askle-pios, or, as the Latins called him, Æsculapius. Among the great healing centres of antiquity his temples were the most famous. Starting as a chthonian deity in Thessaly, he underwent the degradation, to which deities were subject, of being reduced to the rank of a hero, or demi-god, with the peculiarity, however, that his cult was not confined to one spot exclusively. Smitten by the divinizing lightning of Zeus—"Æsculapius ut in deum surgat fulminatur"—the hero was then, by a reverse process, raised to the rank of the Olympian gods, though, like Dionysos, never admitted to the Olympian hall. In his case, as in the case of other chthonian gods, prophecy or divination went hand in hand with healing, and the serpent, too, was sacred to him.[1]

From Thessaly, and with Trikka as the oldest centre, his worship extended not only over Greece, but also to Asia Minor and to Italy. At the time of Alexander the Great the shrines of Asklepios numbered 186, and later 320, while his worship was

[1] Rohde, *Psyche*, 1894, p. 132 f.

23

introduced into Rome in 293 B.C., and was endowed with a temple on the island of the Tiber, which was afterwards taken over by the Church of San Bartolomeo.

But the most famous of all the shrines of "the god of bodily health—*Salvator*, as they called him absolutely"—was at Epidauros in Argos, and the cult there goes back to unknown times. The temple, however, now excavated by the Greek Archæological Society, dates from the fourth century B.C. It consists of a *tholos* or *thymele*, or idealized architectural pit for minor sacrifices, with a labyrinth below (perhaps the home of the sacred serpents), an *abaton* or portico, which was a hospital or *Liegehalle*, open on the south side, with a ward for each sex, four other blocks of buildings opening each on a quadrangle and (on the south of the precinct) a theatre. Within the temple was a great statue of the god in ivory and gold by Thrasymedes, attended by a serpent and dog as his symbols. To this temple the sick resorted from all parts of the Greek world, and its activities continued until they were taken over by the Christian Church, when the god was superseded by the saint.[1]

On the walls of the eastern abaton were placed stone stelæ bearing inscriptions, written by authority, recording cures. These served as instruments of suggestion to patients. Of these cures some are fabulous, some were worked by orthodox methods, and some would come under the head of Spiritual Healing. M. Kavvadias, indeed, is of opinion that

[1] A convenient account of Epidauros is given by Miss Mary Hamilton, *Incubation*, 1906.

up to the Christian era the miracle of cure was wrought in all Asklepieia by prayer. In the inscriptions, however, a repeated feature is the temple-sleep into which the patient was thrown (whether by hypnotism or appropriate drugs is not clear), during which, in vision or in dream, the god appeared and effected the desired cure.

Our knowledge of the process of curing and of the results attained rests on the inscriptions which have been brought to light in the course of the excavations carried on. They are given on large stelæ set up in the porticos, and give forty-four cases of cure. We must recollect, however, that they represent what the officiating priesthood would like said, what the patient would be interested in saying, and that we have no means of checking their accuracy, or of judging what proportion the cures bear to the failures. Nor have we any better method than that of analogy for determining the precise details of the clinic of the operators.

Omitting as irrelevant to our present purposes such stories as describe the restoration of an atrophied eyeball or of a lost head of hair, or the cure of dropsy by cutting off the head, holding up the patient by the heels that the fluid might run out, and the fixing on the head again ; also all other stories of cures which are explicable by ordinary medical science, there remain a number which must be attributed to some form of Spiritual Healing. For example, we have the case of a dumb boy who came as a suppliant to the temple to recover his voice. "When he had performed the preliminary sacrifices and fulfilled the usual rites, the temple priest who bore the sacrificial fire turned to the boy's father and said, 'Do you promise to pay within a year the fees for the cure, if you obtain that for which you have come?' Suddenly the boy answered, 'I do.' His father was greatly astonished at this, and told his son to speak again. The boy repeated the words, and so was cured." With this we may compare the story of the paralytic gentleman in the Neapolitan revolt of 1547, who had himself carried into the square in the arms of his servants, but was found after the tumult on the top of the campanile of San Lorenzo, whither he had climbed. His terror had animated his will, and his will had broken through the bonds, whatever they were, which had prevented his muscles from acting.[1]

This and the case just before cited may be taken, if we may be allowed to anticipate our conclusions, as typical of cases of Spiritual Healing in general. For these belong as a rule (not always) to what the medical faculty is accustomed to describe as "functional," that is, non-organic, or, in other words, to a class of disorders the origin of which cannot be traced to any organic lesion. (For a discussion of the validity of this distinction between functional and organic disease see further, p. 146.)

Another story related on the stelæ is that of Nikanor, a lame man, who, while he was sitting wide awake, had his crutch snatched from him by a boy who, after snatching it, ran away with it. Nikanor got up, ran after the boy, and so was cured. His case may go with the two preceding, or it may

[1] Quoted by Benedetto Croce, *The Philosophy of the Practical*, 1913, p. 175.

go with that of the lame man in *Henry VI*, Part II. Act II. scene i, who found his legs when Gloucester bade the beadle whip him.

Another lame man came to Epidauros on a litter. In his sleep he saw a vision. He thought that the god ordered him to climb a ladder up to the roof of the temple. At daybreak he departed healed. Another man, Kleimenes of Argos, a paralytic, came as a suppliant to the abaton, and in sleep saw a vision of a snake which the god wound round him. The god then took him to a lake, the water of which . . . while he was lying there. . . . "Many men came for that," said the god, "to the sanctuary. He would not do such a thing, but would send him away cured." At daybreak he departed cured. (This inscription is partly erased.)

Another invalid, a sufferer from gout, was walking about in his waking state, when one of the geese in the temple bit his feet, making them bleed, and this cured him.

The other cases tell us of barren women conceiving, wounded men having spear-heads removed, eyesight being restored, an abscess being operated on, facts being revealed in dreams, hair being made to grow, or stone being cured. One story is remarkable, but in the light of our present knowledge not incredible. Pandaros, a Thessalian, had disfiguring marks on his forehead. The god bound them round with a head-band, and on waking it was found that the marks had been transferred to the band. Pandaros afterwards gave some money to a man called Echedoros to present to the god as a thank-offering. When this man went to the god to get healed from similar marks, the god asked him whether he had received from Pandaros any money for an offering, to which he replied that he had not. The god then bound his head as he had bound that of Pandaros, and in the morning Echedoros found that he had not only his own marks, but those of Pandaros as well.

There is, however, one remarkable feature about all, or nearly all, the cures recorded on the stelæ. The temple-sleep plays a leading part. The patient is put to sleep, and during the sleep the cure is effected. In some cases it might be suspected that an anæsthetic drug was used, and that while so "asleep" an operation was performed, as operations undoubtedly were. For example, "a man had an abdominal abscess. He saw a vision, and thought that the god ordered the slaves who accompanied him to lift him up and hold him so that his abdomen could be cut open. The man tried to get away, but the slaves caught him and bound him. So Asklepios cut him open, rid him of the abscess, and then stitched him up again, releasing him from his bonds. Straightway he departed cured, and the floor of the abaton was covered with blood." [1]

Such a story presents no more difficulty than that of any hospital operation of to-day. The only uncertainty is as to the means by which the "sleep" was brought about. Was it by a "miracle," or were drugs used, or hypnotism, or both? And what are we to make of the fact that the inscriptions almost uniformly testify to the instantaneousness of the cure? The next day the patient goes away

[1] The inscriptions recording the cures here tabulated are given in CIG iv. 951-2, but may be more conveniently studied in Hans Lietzmann's *Kleine Texte*, as given in No. 79, *Antike Wundergeschichten*, Bonn, 1911.

cured. But no known drug gives such immediate recovery. On the other hand, even though suggestion given in hypnotic sleep might not actually heal there and then a wound, it might, as is well known, send the sufferer away *believing* that he was healed. And in this way a mental faculty would be brought in to help in the cure, and so the cure would come under the head of Spiritual Healing. But it would seem more rational to assign a "miracle" (in the sense to be discussed later, in Chapter XII) as the cause—that is, an activity of the indwelling Life, which the priests knew how to stimulate when the conditions were favourable.

It is unfortunate that neither Epidauros, nor the temples of Asklepios at Athens or Kos or elsewhere, nor the temple of Amphiaros at Oropos, give us any sure indication of the nature of the "temple-sleep." That it was an invariable part of the therapeutic, that it was preceded by sacrifice and accompanied by dieting, and was also closely connected with divination in some form or other, are facts that are well attested. But more than this we are not told, and we are not justified in inferring more than that the "faith" of the patients was an integral factor in the process by which the cure was brought about. The importance of this factor will appear later. But meanwhile we might be content to say that the healing temples of the Greek world in the four centuries before our era were partly hospitals where surgery and medicine were empirically studied, and partly homes of religion, so that science and faith went hand in hand under the authority of the god exercised by his priest. In later time science dissolved the formal partnership, and so Spiritual Healing became an independent and suspected stranger to orthodox medicine, and remains so to the present time. Whether it might not be worth while for orthodoxy to examine more persistently than it has yet done the modern equivalents of ancient "incubation" is a question for the medical authorities themselves. It is probable that such an investigation would illustrate not only the inscriptions at Epidauros, but the connection between oracle and healings, the functions of the κάτοχοι, or mediums, in the temples of Serapis at Memphis, or of Dionysos at Amphikleia, and the secrecy which hedged in the therapeutic work of Isis in her temple at Tithorea, as described by Pausanias.[1]

A further discussion of this question of the nature and efficacy of the practice of incubation may be deferred until we come to the subject of "Dreams and Spiritual Healing." In Chapter VIII we shall draw attention to the work done by Dr. Sigmund Freud, of Vienna, and by his school in investigating by means of psycho-analysis the hidden psychical ferment which is apt to manifest itself in the phenomena of neurasthenia and hysteria and cognate disorders. And some further examples of incubation will there be given, by way of showing how little there is that is new under the sun, seeing that the same problems emerge again and again in more or less similar forms everywhere and in all ages.

[1] On the general subject of this chapter may be consulted with advantage R. Reitzenstein, *Hellenistische Wundererzählungen*, 1906; O. Weinreich, *Antike Heilungswunder*, 1909, and Dieterich, *Abraxas*, 1891.

CHAPTER III

SPIRITUAL HEALING IN EARLY CHRISTIANITY

WHEN we pass from the Hellenistic world to the Christian we are generally supposed to leave an old world which died for a new world which was then born. The Christ came, we say, crying, "Lo, I make all things new." Yet the contrast is not so sharp as is popularly supposed. The "hard pagan world" did not die, or if it did, it rose again, subsumed in the wonderful institution called the Catholic Church. Indeed (as Tatian assures us), Zeus and Apollo took on the new rôle of "Saviour,"[1] and continued it during the first three Christian centuries. "No one could any longer be a god who was not also a Saviour," says Harnack.[2] The cult of Æsculapius, so far from dying out, seemed almost to have taken a new lease of life, and he became *par excellence* the Saviour, the Θεὸς Σωτήρ. "People betook themselves to his healing centres as they betake themselves to the waters; they invoked him in the illnesses of body and soul; they brought to him, the Saviour-god, the richest presents and dedicated to him their lives."[3]

An unexceptionable testimony to the continued

[1] *Orat.*, 8.
[2] *Mission und Ausbreitung des Christentums*, 1902, p. 78.
[3] *Ibid.*, p. 77.

31

influence of Æsculapius is given by Origen in his
controversy with Celsus, in which the point at issue
is whether Æsculapius or Christ is the real Saviour.
Origen does not see his way to reject the assertion
of Celsus that sicknesses were healed and future
things revealed in all the centres which were dedicated to Æsculapius, as in Epidauros, Trikka, Kos
and Pergamum. Celsus, on the other hand, maintained that many Greeks and barbarians had
actually seen Æsculapius, while all the Christians
saw was a shadow. To which Origen retorts by
pointing to the number of cures effected in the
name of Jesus, and adds that in any case there was
no necessary connection between holiness or virtue
and the power of healing and prophesying. One
thing is clear from the line of argument adopted
by Origen, and that is, that he was not in a position
to deny that Æsculapius was honoured far and
wide as a healing god, and did effect cures.

Into a world full of a passionate desire for salvation from evil both of body and soul the Christ
came. Nor was the longing for escape from bodily
evil less real than the longing to escape from
spiritual evil, and hence the latter was expressed
in terms of the former, as when, for example,
Porphyry describes philosophy as "the saving of
the soul." When, then, Jesus appeared as the Son
of God, it was natural that He should be greeted
as the Great Physician, as the Saviour as well of
body as of mind. The Stoics had prepared the way
for this by their practical doctrines about the "healing and the sickness of the soul," and the close
connection between the two kinds of healing is

shown by the words of Eusebius, in which he says that "Jesus, as a good physician, had, in order to heal the sick, visited that which was abhorrent, and came into touch with that which was loathsome, and Himself felt pain through the sufferings of others."[1]   How tenacious was the belief in Jesus as the healer of bodily sickness appears from the legendary letter of Abgarus, King of Edessa, which saw the light about the middle of the third century, in which he says : "I have heard of thee and thy healings, which thou performest without medicine or drugs. For, as is reported, thou makest the blind to see, the lame to walk, and the lepers to be clean ; thou drivest out unclean spirits and demons, and healest those who were tormented by long-standing sicknesses, and thou awakenest the dead."[2]

This witness rests on the same foundation as do the healing stories of the first three evangelists, and criticism has for several centuries now been busying itself with attempts to discriminate between the different elements which go to compose that foundation.   This is not the place to discuss the theories put out by critics, but it may be said that the tendency is to classify the "miracles" of Jesus into (a) those which are constructed as antitypes to Old Testament typical wonders, as e. g. when Jesus feeds the multitude in the way that Moses did, i. e. "supernaturally"; (b) those which are parables misunderstood and changed into relations of fact, as e. g. the withering of the fig-tree; (c) healings which come under law, even though the precise law be unknown, or half known; and (d) some

[1] H. E., x. 4, 11.   [2] Harnack, *ubi supra*, p. 73.

D

wonders at present inexplicable. We are concerned with the third class only.

The narratives of this class are twofold. In the one case they merely state in general terms that Jesus healed all the sick that were brought to Him out of a whole region, that He healed "all manner of sickness and all manner of disease among the people," or "all sick persons that were taken with divers diseases and torments," or that "great multitudes followed Him and He healed them there." Such statements show both the strength of the tradition that Jesus was a great healer, and also the absence of any detailed knowledge on the part of the evangelist. Hence we are not in a position to infer anything as to the methods of Jesus, or the precise nature of the diseases treated by Him, from statements which are left so vague.

But the second class is more precisely defined. Here we are given, not, indeed, names and dates or references, but what reads like history of actual events. We have stories of demoniacs being cured, stories of paralysis, deafness, blindness, dumbness, curvature, leprosy, flux, fever and dropsy being removed, whether by word or by touch. The three stories of raising the dead to life again stand by themselves, and in no case come under the head of Spiritual Healing.

But are all the others just referred to examples of this method of healing, or must some of them at least be put into another class, and so beyond the scope of these pages? We answer that, in the first place, there is good ground for suspecting that in some cases, e.g. in that of the daughter of the woman of Canaan, of the Gadarene demoniacs, and the dumb man of Matt. ix. 32, the groundwork of the story is the historical fact that the religion of Jesus expelled the worship of idols, and it is significant that in these three cases the sufferer is said to be "demonized," a word of which the most natural meaning is that of being deified, or brought under the power of a demon—that is, of a false god. In other cases, as in that of the man who was lunatic, perhaps that of the blind and dumb man of Matt. xii. 22 (if this, indeed, should not be added to the three above) and others, we have two things: the fact alleged and its interpretation. The evangelist states that a certain man came forward with a specific disease, and he assigns as its cause the action of a demon or an unclean spirit. The difficulty of forming any clinical diagnosis in these cases is caused partly by our not being told enough to enable us to say whether the disease was "functional" or "organic." If the former, we could point to the phenomena of hypnotism since the days of Braid, or to the familiar influence of what we loosely but vividly call a "magnetic personality." In this case we are moving in the familiar ground of natural law.

If the latter were the case, if in any of these instances the disease was "organic," we should be locked up to one or the other of two alternatives. Either we are given a striking example of the power of Life to dominate body, even to the extent of repairing an atrophied organ, a power which we cannot rationally rule out as impossible, though we ought in the name of Truth to view critically the

evidence adduced for any alleged manifestation of
it; or else we must admit the "miraculous," and
so find ourselves in conflict with almost the whole
of modern thought. For that thought, whether in
its scientific or its philosophic form, is admittedly
hostile to any suggestion that Law allows exceptions. If apparent exceptions are alleged, then they
are met with an *a priori* conviction that fuller
knowledge will naturalize them as subjects of Law.

But our present purpose is not concerned with
the philosophical question of "miracles."[1] It is
enough to say that if Life has the power over the
bodily organs which our first alternative suggests,
then its activity comes clearly enough under the
head of Spiritual Healing. If, on the other hand,
the hypothesis of miracles be accepted, the case for
Spiritual Healing is still more cogent. But the
advocate of this power will probably be wise if he
contents himself with the former of these two
alternatives.

There seems, then, no reason why we should rule
out as irrational, when we come to appraise the
Gospel stories of healing, the hypothesis which
explains the *modus operandi* as being determined
by the spiritual order. But this does not absolve
us from the duty of inquiring whether the evangelists are to be followed when they trace the diseases in question to the activity of demons. Or
ought we to say with modern science that our
business is to trace every effect on the physical
plane to a cause on the same plane, and to abstain
from passing over to another class, such as demons

[1] This question will be discussed in Chap. XII.

certainly form? Blindness or deafness, we are told, may be traced to some corruption of an organ, and the decay of that organ may be charted step by step so clearly and certainly that it is an impertinence to drag in a spiritual causality. Demons may exist, or they may not, but in no case is medical science concerned with them, and therefore you may search in vain Gray's *Anatomy*, or Rose and Carless's *Surgery*, for any reference to demons. If the New Testament attributes disease to the activities of demons, so much the worse for it, for it is thereby proved to belong to the pre-scientific period, and, being wrong in this important particular, may very well be an unsafe guide on other points as well.

1. To this we may reply, first, that the ætiology of disease is not quite so simple as this objection would make out. We do not, as a matter of fact, know certainly that physical results flow from physical causes alone. Indeed, we might so far dispute the proposition as to assert that no physical result ever flows from a mere physical cause at all. You may, if you like, say that a blow on the head inflicted by a policeman's bâton is surely of the physical order alone. For was it not physical force measurable in foot-pounds which brought down the piece of wood on my head and broke my skull? Perhaps, but the policeman had some reason for putting out his muscular energy in the precise way he did. He might have been afraid of me, or been commanded by his superior officer to break crowns, or have been intoxicated. Will and purpose cannot be excluded even here, for it is they which direct the application of the force here and now.

Similarly, we shall find, when we look a little closer, that the history of diseases is incomplete when stated in terms of physics alone. For example, I chose when I was younger (what made me so choose may here be neglected) to devote myself to athletics with youthful ardour; this put an undue strain on the muscles of the heart, and their consequent weakness was the forerunner of neurasthenia and dyspepsia. Am I to be told now that my volitions of thirty years ago have no place in the chain of causal events which has made my health what it is? And if not, may it not be that it is not impossible, if only I can find out how, that my volitions may once more be engaged about my health, but now in a wiser way, so as to undo the evil done in youthful ignorance by wiser action prescribed by fuller knowledge? Further, if my own volitions count for something in producing my present physical condition, there seems no valid reason for excluding the volitions of other sentient beings. In other words, if there be indeed demons, their volitions, too, may have to be taken into account in a thoroughgoing diagnosis.

2. There is good reason for the belief that all change proceeds from a spiritual force. As Kant has taught us, the principle of Causality is one of the *a priori* forms of our Understanding. But this principle is not necessarily *a priori* in the sense that it is prior to all experience, but in the sense that it is now prior to all possible experience. "It is plainly enough derived," says Lotze, "from experience of our own activity, and the contrast of the living nature that acts and the lifeless thing that

suffers."[1] So our language, with its main gram-
matical division into substantives for things, adjec-
tives for qualities, and verbs for actions, would not
be possible "unless they had been preceded in
consciousness by the contrast between the Subject
and Object of actions—the usual form of the
common notion of Cause." It is the experience
of willing which gives us the concept of change,
and hence the movement. Hence, if we detect
changes in our bodily conditions, it is not rational
to seek to account for them by previous changes of
the same physical order; we are acting rationally
only when we trace them back to spirit in some
form. And if no incarnate spirit can be found or
suspected, it is again rational to inquire whether
some non-incarnate spirit—we do not say bodiless
—may not be the efficient cause of the change we
are trying to account for. But this would introduce
the possibility of demons.

3. It is true that no proof, or even evidence, has
been produced for the existence and the activity of
demons, and for the good reason that neither is,
perhaps, possible. All we can say is that their
non-existence is more improbable than their existence. For on any theistic theory of the world, or,
indeed, on any idealistic, there is no sufficient
reason for limiting the *nous*, or reason, at the back
of things to the human horizon, for supposing that
the capabilities of the world are exhausted by mankind. Moreover, just as the ordinary matter we
are acquainted with can and does exist in a threefold degree of density, so in all probability may

[1] *Microcosmus*, i. 677.

animated bodies. And the "psychical" body we bear now may be indefinitely transcended by finer and finer bodies, just as it is not inconceivable that it may in its turn transcend indefinitely many lower orders of bodies. In other words, it is only our racial conceit which makes us assume that the bodies we are familiar with are the only bodies in the world. But if there be others, we have no good ground for assigning them to "good spirits" only. Evil spirits may well be as integral a part of the existing order as good ones, and, in fact, what we know of that order gives force to the argument from analogy that evil spirits are posited in the cosmic order together with good spirits.

4. An argument of a different character, and one on which too great reliance must not be placed, may be drawn from the phenomena of cancer; and it is mentioned here because claims have been made, though not, so far as the writer is aware, been substantiated, for the cure of cancer by spiritual means. All that is known of cancer is that "certain cells, which are apparently of a normal character and have previously performed normal functions, begin to grow and multiply in an abnormal way in some part of the body. They continue this process so persistently that they first invade and then destroy the surrounding tissues; nothing can withstand their march. They are, moreover, carried to other parts of the body, where they establish themselves and grow in the same way."[1] Now the singular thing at present about cancer, apart from its

[1] See R. Tanner-Hewlett, *Pathology General and Special*, 1906, Chap. III.

horrible "malignancy," is that, in spite of the work of the Imperial Cancer Research Fund in England, and of similar bodies in Germany and the United States, no theory of the origin of the disease holds the field. All that has been done is to clean the slate of the many conjectures which have been popularized, and to trace more clearly the growth of the disease. But, looking to the fact that cancer is abnormal cell-proliferation, and that the cell is the simplest form through which Life functions, the conjecture—it is little more—may be hazarded that where physical nature affords no way out psychical nature may help. As the proportion per million living persons in England and Wales of deaths from cancer has risen from 445 forty years ago to 861 now, and as cancer is a disease of older years, that is, when the life-force is least master in its own house, it is not improbable that the origin and cure of cancer should be looked for in the "soul" rather than in the body. And the cases of what medical science describes as "spontaneous cures" may be accounted for by some untracked healthy activity of the Life within. These considerations do not in any way affect directly the question about the existence and activity of demons, but they may indirectly affect it by strengthening the belief in the potentialities of Life, and, therefore, the belief in more manifestations of it than are recorded in ordinary experience.

Hence, without prejudging for or against the hypothesis which attributes diseases, or at all events some diseases, to the agency of demons, we shall be content for the present to leave the question

open. As to the method of healing, however (apart
from the question of the origin of the disease),
which appears in the Gospel story, no other hypothesis meets the facts as they are there presented
but that which assigns them to Spiritual Healing.

In saying this we are aware that we are likely
to be accused of trying to explain *ignotum per
ignotius*, the familiar by the unfamiliar. Blindness
we know, and paralysis we know, but Spiritual
Healing we do not know. The objection is just,
but all that can be said in answer to it here is that
at present it is being used in a negative sense to
cover some therapeutic activity which does not come
under drugs, diet, exercise, massage or the knife,
under the ordinary instruments of orthodox medicine. Later on we shall endeavour to supply a
positive content to the term Spiritual Healing. All
we are concerned with for the moment is the fact—
for it would be foolish to extend our scepticism to
this fact—that Jesus was believed to work cures
and did work cures, and that as He spake with
authority and not as the scribes, so He healed by
some kind of spiritual action and not as the
physicians of the day.

With one exception, little is added to our knowledge of Spiritual Healing by the New Testament
outside the four Gospels. The beliefs of the
Apostolic Age about its powers are summed up
in the current ending of St. Mark's Gospel, where
it is said that Christians were endowed with power
to cast out devils, to speak with fresh tongues, to
tread on serpents, to be immune from poisons, and
to heal by the laying on of hands. Peter raised

Tabitha from death through prayer, as earlier his word had committed to death Ananias and Sapphira. His shadow, even, was thought to have healing power, just as handkerchiefs or aprons carried away from Paul's body caused diseases to depart from the sick at Ephesus. It is difficult to say how much of the repeated statements in general terms in the Acts of the Apostles is due to rhetoric, how much is symbolic, and how much is based on specific acts of Spiritual Healing. But it would be carrying scepticism too far to brush aside the whole belief in supernormal powers exercised by the early Church as being due to credulity or superstition. The general picture of exaltation due to the possession of extraordinary powers must have some basis of fact, though the fact is not necessarily of the miraculous order. We must recollect that Christianity was the ending of the formal side of an older order, and was essentially the opening of the flood-gates of "æonian life," and that, therefore, the wonder would have been, not that it accomplished things which seemed miraculous, but that it did not. So far we may safely trust the narrative, even after all deductions have been made for bias, for the author's remoteness from the time of the history, and for imperfection of critical method.

What is given as history in the Acts of the Apostles appears as theory in the Epistles. Writing to the Corinthians, St. Paul refers to certain supernormal powers he calls gifts which he speaks of almost as being normal in the Christian community. Among them he includes "gifts of healing." What their precise nature was, their limits or their frequency, he does not say. He is content to say that they were a gift from the same Spirit from whom all gifts come, and we are led to suspect that they were connected with the rite of laying on of hands, the original meaning of which seems to have been forgotten at a very early date. We shall have something to say about it later on.

It was the fashion in the pre-critical period of the study of Christian origins, say a generation ago, to bring the "miracles" of the New Testament down to the close of the Apostolic Age, and to treat all subsequent "miracles" as marked by fraud or credulity. Protestantism, indeed, has never been quite easy on the field of mediæval wonders, and its theory of miracles blinded it to the true meaning of the historical in the New Testament itself. It claimed, in accordance with its principle, that so long as the Apostles lived, or at the outside so long as the disciples of the Apostles lived, "miracles" were common, but as men moved further away from the days of Jesus Christ they lost more and more of the power of working miracles, until at last it died out. Anyhow, after the end of the second century no more "miracles" are to be accepted.

Certainly in that period the claim to healing powers was constantly made. Justin Martyr asserts against Trypho "the mighty deeds that now take place in the power of His name," and later on he specifically mentions "healing" as among the gifts which disciples receive as they are worthy.[1] He again affirms that demons were exorcised in his day

[1] *Dial.*, Chap. XXXIX.

in the name of Jesus Christ.[1] And in his Second Apology he says that "numberless demoniacs throughout the whole world and in your city (Rome) many of our Christian men exorcising them in the name of Jesus Christ, who was crucified under Pontius Pilate, have healed and do heal, rendering helpless and driving the possessing devils out of the men, though they could not be cured by the other exorcists and those who used incantations and drugs."[2]

The gift of prophecy which ordinarily accompanies the gift of healing had not died out in the Apostolic Age, as Montanism later testifies, and now and then the claim is made that the dead were raised up, but the claim never rests on actual observation or on accredited testimony, but on hearsay only. Moreover, it is not impossible that the exorcism of devils is but the negative side of "Baptism into the Name," through which the worship of "devils"—that is, of idols—was definitely ended for the baptized person. So that, on the whole, we are left in a state of some uncertainty about the facts of Spiritual Healing alike in the time of the New Testament and that which immediately followed it. All we can say, and this we can safely say, is that the first age of the Church was an age of spiritual exaltation and spaciousness, of enlarged consciousness and deepened faith and more buoyant hope, and that it supplied, therefore, the conditions out of which Spiritual Healing might be fairly expected, judging by analogy, to take its rise. The presumption is in favour of such healing

[1] *Dial.*, Chap. LXXXV.   [2] ii. *Apol.*, c. 6.

arising. Whether it is more than a presumption will depend on whether the evidence from other quarters supports it or neutralizes it. And yet it would be unreasonable to deny that Jesus did perform acts of Spiritual Healing just because the evidence for its character in detail is elusive. Even if we are pointed to the facility with which wonders accumulate round great personalities so as to succeed in clothing them with a nimbus of legend, we are still justified in retorting that this very process presupposes, at all events, the greatness of the personality. And if Apollonius of Tyana be dragged in to discredit the gospel narrative, we may say that, unless we are tied to some artificial theory of miracles, there is no reason why Apollonius should not have been a wonder-worker, even if we were to accept the hypothesis that his story was deliberately concocted for the purpose of supplying a pagan antidote for the Christian propaganda.

CHAPTER IV

SPIRITUAL HEALING IN THE MIDDLE AGE

THE history of Spiritual Healing in the later Christian centuries, say, from the Peace of the Church in A.D. 313 to the Reformation which began to be active in the sixteenth century, will, many will urge, add but little to our knowledge of Spiritual Healing. Its merit will be of a negative character as supplying an object lesson in the need of cautious criticism, if we are not to be led astray by our fancies. For nowhere more than here is the maxim exemplified, "Omne ignotum pro magnifico," and at few times has there been a greater disposition to believe what we want to believe than nowadays, when a quickened sense of the evil of all disease makes us impatient of its existence, and ready to take short cuts to its removal. Hence a short study of the "age of faith" may have a steadying effect on our judgment of claims to healing powers so frequently made in our hearing to-day. But, on the other hand, we may find ultimately that lurking in the myths and legends of the Middle Age there is a valuable residuum of solid fact.

We must recollect that miracles in the strict sense of the word, that is, as arbitrary interferences with the order of Nature, were in the air during the Middle Age, and that, therefore, they might be expected at any moment to occur. With this supposition so deeply rooted, the wonder would be if miracles did not happen, and the truth seems to be that they became so common as to cease to be miracles. Every saint was a wonder-worker, and many were wonder-workers who were not saints. What Mgr. Guérin says of St. William is typical of most saints: "Without troubling the elements he subdued the rigid laws of Nature. A dying infant he restored full of life and energy to his delighted mother. His benediction unlocked the limbs of a paralytic. To a possessed person he gave peace of mind and body. He broke a prisoner's chains. By the mere touch of his hand the blind, the deaf, the dumb recovered the use of their senses." Even after his death another eulogist declared that by his tombstone "diseases and mortal wounds were cured, demoniacs were set free, lunatics recovered their reason, the dumb spoke, the deaf heard, the blind saw, prisons were opened, chains fell away, infants carried off by wolves were found again, safe and sound." We seem to catch an echo in these and similar expressions of the vague generalization of a Justin and a Tertullian, but we can hardly conclude more than that St. William was a remarkable man who did some remarkable things, and was credited with more.

The life of St. Carlo Borromeo may again be taken as typical, and the miracles ascribed to him are recited in the bull of his canonization. The following are some of them. By his prayers he healed of mortal illness an archbishop of Matia who had been given up by his physicians. His making the sign of the Cross saved an abbot and his companion from being drowned in the Ticino. His prayer saved from death another man whose horse had thrown him over a precipice. His manual benediction drove a crowd of devils out of a young man. He instantaneously cured a double tertian ague of eight months' standing. He healed a lady of a disease caused by witchcraft. Nor was his power lessened by death. Being invoked when dead, he cured in an instant, on the feast of St. John the Baptist, 1601, a man who had been paralysed for eight and a half years. Similarly, he removed two tumours from the eyes of a boy, and restored his sight. He appeared to a certain Martha Vighia of Milan, whose sight had been entirely destroyed, in her sleep, and bade her visit his tomb. She did so, kissed his tombstone, and saw. A man suffering from scrofula also visited the saint's tomb, invoked him, and went away whole.

Is there any essential difference between these wonders and those written down on the stelæ at Epidauros?

St. Germanus, Bishop of Paris in the sixth century, was a famous spiritual healer, and was "an apostolic man, the father, the physician, the shepherd and the love of his people." When he went to church the sick were placed in a double row for him to heal them. "The straw of his bed, the fragments and threads of his robe, his saliva, his tears, his words, the water in which he washed

E

his hands, his look, his touch, his dreams during
sleep, each and all carried miraculous remedies."
The life of St. Vincent Ferrier is more wonderful
than most. He was almost a professional miracle-
worker. A "miracle-bell" was rung every morning when he began his healing work. As Mgr.
Guérin says : "Had he, in the course of those
twenty years, performed only eight miracles daily,
the number would amount to the number of
58,400. But this is an under-estimate, since it is
an ascertained fact that our saint performed them
not only in the public assemblies and while teaching, but while walking, stopping at home, at every
moment, we may say. Hence the writers of his
Life are wont to say : ' It was a miracle when he
performed no miracles '; the greatest miracle he
wrought was to work none."

St. Francis of Paula is only second to St.
Vincent Ferrier in the range and activity of his
thaumaturgic powers. Leaving out of account the
stories in which he figures as moulding the world
around him at his will, it was stated at the process
of his canonization that he was known to have
healed as many as a hundred persons in one day,
and that he was always healing, and with such
success that he certainly held in his hands the keys
of life and death. "He gave eyes to the blind,
hearing to the deaf, speech to the dumb; he made
the halt to walk, the cripple to have the use of
his limbs; and he recalled six persons to life. One
man, even, he brought back to life twice." To
quote again Mgr. Guérin : "Lepers, dropsical,
paralytics, people afflicted with stone, gravel, colic,

indigestion and every kind of illness, outbreak or tumour found in his charity instantaneous relief. Never was there any illness, however great or incurable it might seem, which could withstand his voice or his touch."

Another saint who may be brought forward as a witness to tell us what wonders pervaded the age of faith is St. Geneviève. The same authority thus describes her marvels: "At the Church of St. Denis was a lamp whose oil was never consumed, though it was burning continually, and though it was being frequently drawn from in order to the healing of the sick.[1] From it the blind received their sight, the dumb the use of their tongue, possessed persons deliverance, those suffering from fever immediate and complete health. One woman who was rebuked for working on our Lady's birthday had replied impudently that the Virgin was a poor woman like herself, and in punishment for this blasphemy her fingers stuck so tight to the comb with which she was carding wool that they could not be separated from it. She was, however, cured when she prayed near the tomb. One day the Seine strangely overflowed its banks and flooded all the churches and houses near it to the depth of several storeys, when they found the bed on which St. Geneviève had given up her spirit surrounded by the water as by a wall, without being submerged or even damped. Then the flood ceased, and the river returned to its bed. At the time of Louis the Fat there arose in Paris a cruel sickness called by the

[1] See note on p. 62.

doctors the feu sacré, or cancerous and epidemic form of erysipelas. Many died of it without any cure being found. This compelled the clergy and laity to have recourse to St. Geneviève. All the poor feverous patients were thereupon cured at once with the exception of three, who lacked faith, or whom God did not will to cure for some unknown reason. The whole of France was wont to implore her assistance in time of war, pestilence, famine, drought, flood, excessive rain, and in every time of need. Wars have been ended, pestilences banished, dryness turned to rain and vice versâ, and barren land made fruitful. This was experienced in the year 1675, when through continuous rain all hope of harvest had been abandoned, and afterwards a sudden and mar- vellous change brought about an abundance such as had not before been seen." [1]

Perhaps it may be well to describe in a little fuller detail the doings of a few of the more popular saints of the ages which saw the full secular glory of the Catholic Church, because their very popularity is sufficient testimony to the fact that they were faithful reflections of the beliefs and expectations of the folk. And those folk- beliefs, we must recollect also, were of pagan origin, and remained pagan in all but in name. We shall select three pairs of wonder-working saints and three single workers : viz. for the first, Cosmas and Damian, Cyrus and John, Protasius and Gervasius; and for the second, St. Thomas of Canterbury, St. Ubaldo and St. Martin of Tours.

[1] Guérin, *Vies des Saints*, 1880, i. 100 f.

Cosmas and Damian

The most interesting of all mediæval saints to those interested in Spiritual Healing are Cosmas and Damianus, "brothers, physicians, 'silverless,' martyrs. These four facts are all that can be said to be known about them, and though they supply little to amuse the mind, they afforded much to feed the heart of Christendom."[1] The epithet "silverless,"*ἀνάργυροι,*was given to those physicians who took no fees, but were content to bring their patients to Christ through the signs of healing wrought by them. Of the three pairs of brothers, Cosmas and Damian, the Roman, the Arabian and the Asiatic, known to the Greek Church, and celebrated by it on July 1, October 17, and November 1 respectively, the second are the best known, principally because they alone are recognized in the west.[2] The Latin Church observes September 27 as the day of their martyrdom. This second pair were twins, born in Arabia, and practised the art of healing in the seaport of Ægea, on the Gulf of Iskanderun in Cilicia. During the persecution of Diocletian they were first tortured

---

[1] E. H. Birks, in Smith's *Dict. of Chr. Biog.*, 1877, i. 691.

[2] The three pairs are probably the outcome of three festivals and not *vice versâ.* " Diese Vervielfältigung der beiden Heiligen ist naturlich unrichtig und erklärt sich aus ihren verschiedenen Festen" (Ehrhard, *Rom. Quartalschr.*, xi. 1897, S. 109, 1). But though the West celebrates the Arabs, Deubner (*Kosmas und Damian*, Leipzig, 1907) has given good reason for his view that neither the Arabian nor the Roman pair was original, but the Asiatic, and that the martyrs rose out of the form of the "doctors and veterinaries," and the wonder-workers out of the martyrs.

ineffectively by the prefect Lysias, and then beheaded. Their remains were buried in the city of Cyrus in Syria, and in the sixth century the Emperor Justinian restored the city in their honour, and after being himself cured of a dangerous illness by their intercession, he rebuilt their church at Constantinople. About the same time Pope Felix IV erected a church at Rome in their honour, in which the art remains are still famous.

But it is hazardous to endorse this history as being sufficiently authenticated, and all we are justified in saying is that the very uncertainty of the legends of these two saints affords a presumption that they rest on earlier pagan legends of a similar character. And this seems to be confirmed by the appearance of other pairs of healing saints such as St. Pantaleon (afterwards called Panteleemon because of the grace vouchsafed to his prayer), a martyr and physician of Nicomedia, associated with Hermolaus, who converted him to Christ,[1] or as John and Cyrus, of whom John was a soldier of rank at the time of Diocletian, and was associated in the legends of martyrdom with Cyrus, a physician of Alexandria.[2]

---

[1] *Acta SS.*, July 27, Boll. vol. xxxiii. p. 397 ff.

[2] The Bollandist relates that Cyrus, "on becoming a monk, changed his mode of healing, and thenceforth neither was, nor was thought to be a physician, but rather a worker of miracles." John was from Edessa, a fact not altogether without point when taken in conjunction with the references of Epiphanius to the two wonder-working saints in the remark, when he mentions Edessa, that "there are buried Cyrus and John." The Acts of the two saints tell us that in the time of Theodosius, Cyril of Alexandria, in order to expel Isis from Menuthis, went in search of the bones of the two saints, and finding them in the church of St. Mark, translated them to Menuthis in great pomp, and so

Another pair of wonder-workers meet us in Florus and Laurus, whose sacred day is August 18. Their story is as follows: They were taught stone-cutting by the martyrs Patroclus and Maximus. From Byzantium they went in search of work to Ulpiana, a city in Dardania. The governor Lycon, to whom they applied, sent them to Licinius, the son of Queen Elpidia. Licinius commissions them to build him a temple after his own plans, and he supplies them with the necessary funds. These they spend on the poor, but work by day on the temple, and spend their nights in prayer. The angels, however, help them in the work, and so the temple is at length finished. Merentius, the chief priest of the temple, becomes a Christian on his son Athanasius being cured of blindness by the two saints. The temple is then consecrated as a Christian church, and the idols are destroyed. Licinius, on hearing of this malfeasance, first burns alive all the poor who had been given his money in charity, flays alive Florus and Laurus, and then sends them to Lycon, who throws them into a dry well, where they die. Afterwards their bones are recovered, and, as was usual in such cases, they work miracles. Now Prof. Rendel Harris has pointed out that whereas the Greek Church honours Florus and Laurus on August 18, the Roman Church honours on that day St. Helena. He hence suggests that Florus and Laurus are a Christian mask for

---

drove out the heathen goddess. See *Acta Sanct.*, Jan. 31, vol. iii. p. 696 ff.

Castor and Pollux, whose sister was Helena, and that they may be also paralleled by the Dioscuri of Thebes, Amphion and Zethus, to whom the Emperor Tiberius erected two pillars at Antioch, similar to those at Hierapolis and Edessa. With Florus and Laurus may be also compared the Milan martyrs, Protasius and Gervasius, and, above all, the widely-popular Cosmas and Damian.

It is not to our present purpose to dwell on the general community of functions of these allied heavenly beings. The Açvins of the Vedas, the Dioscuri, the sons of Antiope, Florus and Laurus, Jude-Thomas, Protasius and Gervasius betake themselves from time to time to dispelling darkness, helping in battle, healing the sick, helping in sex-matters, saving at sea, mastering horses, making ploughs, or building.[1] It is enough to show that healing was practised by them, and that no difference in principle exists between the healing effected by the pagan hero and that effected by the Christian saint.

Among other beneficent works the Dioscuri were also healing gods. Thus a certain Phormio, being wounded at Sagra, was healed of his wound in Sparta after he had invoked them. Hesychius Milesius relates that in the temple of the Dioscuri at the altar of Semester, constructed at the junction of the rivers, there took place for men a dismissal of sufferings. And a scholium speaks of the twins as having told oracularly at night of the conquest and capture of Perses, King of Macedonia, and

[1] See the table in J. Rendel Harris, *The Dioscuri in the Christian Legends*, 1903, p. 61.

adds that in their temples they were wont to give interpretations of dreams. So, too, when once the Roman people were suffering from a pestilence, Castor and Pollux appeared in dreams, and told them how they might be cured of their disease.[1]

The evidence that Cosmas and Damian took over the healing activities of Castor and Pollux is sufficient. In the ninth *Wunder* printed by Deubner[2] it is expressly related that the Greeks were in the habit of sending, when ill, to Castor and Pollux for help; for "how could they have sent, as they should have done, to Cosmas and Damian, seeing that they were ignorant of the Lord of these and of all men, our Lord Jesus Christ, who heals every disease and all weakness through His saints Cosmas and Damian?" However, these latter, on being visited by the Greek suppliant, did their wonted work of healing so well that Castor and Pollux were clearly shown to be inferior to Cosmos and Damian, and were compelled to give place, and the orthodox and genuine faith of the Christians stood out as being that which gave health and strength. Peter of Argos has a notable sentence in which he says: "Who shall tell the mighty acts of the Lord or show forth all His praises? For men no longer run to the demons, the deceivers of the people, and to their wooden images, their carved statues, and to the ignorance of their ambiguous oracles; they no longer have recourse to the Dioscuri, and the

[1] Pauly, *Realencyclopädie*, s. v. vol. v. pt. I. col. 1097. Myriantheus, *Açvins*, conjectures that the warrior physicians Machaon and Podaleirios were originally Thessalian Dioscuri.

[2] *Kosmas und Damian*, Leipzig, 1907, p. 113 ff.

Cheirons and the Asklepii when they are suffering from illnesses and beg for healing from them, but they fly to the Lord of all as the healer of bodies and souls through his 'silverless' saints."[1]

The Bollandists give several lists of miracles attributed to these saints, distinct from the list which they head as "partim fabulosa, partim incerta." It is to be noted that the miracles of healing attributed to them were performed through their relics, and that therefore the date is irrelevant to their genuineness. Under the auspices of Maximilian, Count Palatine of the Rhine, relics of SS. Cosmas and Damian were translated from the metropolitan church of Bremen to the temple of Michael the Archangel in Munich, and the accounts of the miracles there performed are, as the Bollandists proudly assert, contemporaneous and carefully selected. Two youths, one struck down with a sudden fever, and one with a dangerous "frenzy," and both beyond help from their doctors, were healed in answer to their prayers. A cripple who could not walk without crutches offered a candle at the altar of the saints, and was then able to walk. Others were cured of trouble in the feet, of blindness, of lunacy. A member of the Elector's family owed her life to the saints, after receiving the viaticum and the holy oil. One of the Jesuit priests of the church, suddenly seized with diarrhœa the night before he was to deliver an annual funeral oration for the Elector Maximilian, was cured by prayer to the saints, and so enabled to deliver his oration. A

[1] Deubner, *ut supra*, p. 57.

very worthy man, while picking his teeth, was so careless as to swallow the toothpick, and was saved from being choked by the two heavenly physicians, who gradually caused the intrusive pick to move. The proof of the miracle was to be seen in the perpetual light before the altar which the patient's gratitude supplied. Indeed, so renowned became the altar where the two heavenly physicians practised that some 860 outside priests celebrated there. In 1655 a girl was cured of an affection of one eye which threatened the loss of both; in the next two years no cure is recorded, but in 1658 both a man and his beast obtained relief. Another man was cured by the saints of arthritis; but when he omitted to pay what he had promised, the arthritis returned, and was only expelled by the saints on his fulfilling his promises. A woman, too, was cured of a withered hand and arm, whereupon she made her *ex voto* offering.

A church dedicated to the two saints existed at Kaufbeuren in Bavaria, and there, between the years 1628 and 1670, such miraculous cures as the following took place. A churchwarden recovered his sight. The librarian was cured of three fatal tumours through the piety of his wife. A knight recovered from the bite of a venomous snake. His children bring back from the brink of the grave a man named John Geiger, suffering from creeping insanity. Maria Schollhorin had a tumour removed miraculously of the size of an egg. Maria Kocherin could not be cured by any "acatholic" of a stubborn swelling in the knee; the saints cured her in return for a white wax candle. Philip Magg was delivered from hernia, and Joannes Unsin, whose shoulder-bone had been broken by the fall on it of an oak-tree, went away from the saints' altar whole. John Eschelauer was doubly blessed. The saints removed a tumour from his daughter's breast and restored his horse to its former strength. John Miller's daughter was cured of insomnia which had troubled her for a fortnight. Ignatius Hauderer, a child of seven years, lame and bent from his birth, became quite strong and well after being brought to the saints by his parents. Maria Konigman had two daughters, one suffering for six weeks from general debility, and one from goitre. The saints healed both. Christian Most of Upper Bavaria, George Lieb of Frisinga, and several other rustics vow, with a gift to the saintly patrons, their horses infected with a pestilence and without all doubt about to die. The horses, however, are completely cured.

One or two observations on these excerpts from the wonderful doings related of Cosmas and Damian will be enough. No difference exists between the wondrous cures wrought by pagan gods such as Asklepios and those wrought by these Christian saints. No distinction is made between organic and functional disorders. The conduct of the saints when defrauded of the offerings promised to them is exactly the same as that of Asklepios in similar circumstances. In pagan and Christian temples alike *ex voto* offerings are intimately connected with the cures effected. No boundary, such as later science has drawn between man and lower animals, is allowed to interfere with the saints' wonder-working power. Like the God of the psalmist, they save both man and beast. If we accept the stories of cures effected by the Christian saint we can hardly reject the like stories of cures proceeding from pagan heroes or gods. The two saints appear to be Castor and Polydeuctes in a Christianized form.[1] Many of the wonders worked by the saints in the seventeenth century are particularized, and are not to be rejected as inventions merely because their nature is unusual, any more than they are to be attributed as of necessity to the two saints. The Bollandists exercised some discretion in what they have admitted, but we are in a better position than they for estimating the value to be assigned to the wonders they relate.[2] Lastly, it is to be noted that the practice of incubation is rarely mentioned in the *Acta* in connection with Cosmas and Damian.

CYRUS AND JOHN

The home of these wonder-working saints was at Menuthis in Egypt near to Canopus. There was their tomb, a sacred fountain and a temple in their

[1] Alfred Maury, *Rev. archeol.*, vi. 1849, 161, thinks that the two saints took over the work of Asklepios, and builds this on the supposed existence of a temple of that god at Ægea, where the two Arabian martyrs were celebrated. But, after all, Asklepios was not the only healing god in the Greek world. "The Servians call Kosmas and Damian *vratchi*, soothsayers, physicians. . . . . In the legend of Crescentia, Peter, like a second Woden, appears as an old man, conducts the heroine back from the rock in the sea, and endows her with the gift of healing, or himself heals." Grimm, *Teut. Mythol.*, iv. 170, 2.

[2] *Acta Sanctorum*, vol. xlvii. p. 400 ff. ; September 27.

honour. Their wondrous deeds are recorded in the
Encomium of the Blessed Sophronius, afterwards
Bishop of Jerusalem.[1] He says that he himself
had recourse to the two saints for the curing of an
infection of the eyes, and on beholding the abundance of miracles performed in their basilica, he was
fired with a desire to know more about them, but
could find to his amazement but little, and so was
led to provide Christian truths to take the place of
legends about pagan gods. In the course of his
encomium we learn that incubation was practised,
and the saints appeared in sleep to their devotees
and instructed them in dreams. Sometimes the
dreams became effective in the morning only. The
saints heal by the laying on of hands—they would
touch the eyes of the sick man, and so heal him
without drugs. Or they healed through the application of the holy oil taken from the lamp kept
burning in their temple.[2] They would appear suddenly, and with garments bright and glistening,
or in the garb of the monk, and sometimes were
seen by those asleep outside the church.

[1] Migne, *Pat. series Gr.*, vol. lxxxvii. pars iii. cols. 3379–
3696.
[2] " Oil found in the tombs of saints, or even that which was
taken from lamps which burned before their shrines, has been
anciently often used with devotion as a relick. . . . St. Gregory
the Great sent to Queen Theodilinda the oils, as he calls them,
of SS. Peter, Paul, and of nearly seventy other martyrs and
confessors at Rome; and some portions called the oil of many
hundreds and others of many thousands (see Muratoni, *Anec.
Lat.*, t. 2; Mabillon, *Diss. des SS. inconnus*, c. 19, p. 103, and
App. p. 174). Paul Warnefrid (*De Gest. Longob.*, 1, 2, c. 15)
attributes a miraculous healing of sore eyes to the application
of oil taken from a lamp burning before St. Martin's altar."
Alban Butler, *Lives of the Saints*, vol. xi. p. 227 n.

Sophronius (died about A.D. 636), besides writing the encomium of Cyrus and John, also compiled a record of seventy of their miracles, being moved to this number, as he says, by mystical considerations. Among them are found the healing of persons afflicted with obstinate constipation, fistula, cataract, gout, leprosy, demoniacal possession, impotence, cancer, dropsy, blindness. A girl was saved from being hurt by a fall from a height. Another, named Theodora, was made to vomit a frog which she had swallowed. Dorothea's son Callinicus had swallowed a serpent's egg, and the egg had produced a serpent which wriggled about within and tortured him. But the saints, on being appealed to, sent the mother-serpent who had laid the egg, and she, gliding about among the suppliants and hissing, the young serpent at last heard his mother's sibilation and came forth, to the great honour of Cyrus and John. The last of the miracles which Sophronius records was performed on himself, an operation for cataract. Cyrus, habited as a monk, appeared to him with John, who was clothed in the robes of Peter, the pretorian prefect. John asked Cyrus if he had a disciple named Homer, and when Cyrus said he had none so named, then the two saints agreed that it was God who was healing Sophronius and also warning him by this figurative expression to be careful not to fall into the mental blindness of the pagan poet.[1]

How little there is that is new under the sun is

<hr>

[1] See Deubner, *De Incubatione*, pp. 80-98, and Sophronius in Migne, *ut supra*, cols. 3123-3676.

shown by one of the miracles ascribed to the saints of which Christodorus, "œconomus" of the Church, was the hero. This man, sailing once on the lake Mareia on his way to Marcotis, was overtaken by a sudden storm of which the waves threatened to swamp his boat. He feared that he would become the food of fishes even if he escaped the jaws of the crocodiles, but bethought himself of invoking the saints. They, hearing his prayer, came at once to his succour, "since no distance stands in the way of their coming and their health-giving protection, no land or lake or sea, no place that is near, none that is far off, but everywhere, whosoever may have invoked them, him they immediately come to and help and save and protect. Whether it be an attack of spiritual foes, there they plunge into the fight and bring about a victory on behalf of him who has invoked them; or whether it be an attack made by wicked men or of beasts, they give their help. So also they assuage the sharpest and most intolerable pains of disease and act as kindly physicians. Or if there be danger at sea or on a lake, as in the case of Christodorus, they still the winds and cause the waves to subside." [1] This passage of Sophronius lets us see clearly that Cyrus and John had stepped into the place formerly occupied by Castor and Polydeuctes.

PROTASIUS AND GERVASIUS

These twin-saints are interesting if only for their appearing in the history of St. Ambrose, and

[1] Migne, *Pat. series Gr.*, vol. lxxxvii. pars iii. col. 3438.

there manifesting their power in the recovery of sight for a blind man. St. Ambrose was desirous of finding some relics to give added dignity to a magnificent church he was about to consecrate at Milan. He therefore ordered excavations to be made in the Church of St. Nabor and St. Felix near their tomb. There, to be sure, were soon discovered the bodies of "two men of wondrous size, such as ancient times produced," together with much fresh blood, the "miraculous token of martyrdom," says Cardinal Newman. The relics were removed to the Church of St. Fausta and then to the new basilica, where Ambrose delivered some highly rhetorical harangues. "Old men remembered that they had heard formerly the names of these martyrs—Gervasius and Protasius—and had read the title on their grave. Miracles crowded thick upon one another. They were mostly cures of demoniacs and of sickly persons; but one blind man received his sight. . . . Ambrose himself eagerly and positively affirms the reality of the cure; and Augustine, who generally held that the age of miracles was past, also bears witness to the common acceptance of the fact at Milan. . . . The Arians, as we learn from Ambrose and Paulinus, made light of the healing of demoniacs, and were sceptical about the blind man's history."[1] The fact seems to be that the blind man, a butcher, named Severus, whose blindness was said to have been removed by merely touching the pall that covered the sacred relics, was cured or partially cured by

[1] J. Ll. Davies, in Smith's *Dict. of Christ. Biol.*, s. v. Ambrosius, p. 96.

F

what we now call faith-healing.[1] He at all events
ceased to pursue his calling, and spent his time for
the remainder of his life in the church in some
subordinate capacity.

St. Thomas of Canterbury

Thomas was murdered on December 29, 1170,
and almost immediately afterwards miracles began
to be worked in connection with the saint. It is
significant that it was among the poor that the
stories of these miracles originated, and that it was
they who provided the patients who sought, or
perhaps even demanded, healing. The last to be
convinced of the saint's power were the aristocracy,
the prelates, the barons and the king. One of the
most extraordinary acts of Spiritual Healing performed by the saint was the healing of Eilward,
which is so instructive that it deserves quoting in
full. The following is the account given by
Benedict, a monk (afterwards prior) of Canterbury.

"There was one of the common folk, Eilward by
name, in the king's town of Weston in the county
of Bedford. One of his neighbours, Fulk, owed
him a *denarius* as part of rent for cornland, and
put off payment on the excuse of not having the
money. One day, a holiday, when they were going
to the ale-house together, as is the English custom,

---

[1] This is the inference Dr. Abbott draws from the assertion of
the Arians preserved by Ambrose. He says : "Negant esse eum
illuminatum, sed ille non negat se sanatum. . . . Isti beneficium
negant qui factum negare non possunt." Something they
admitted had taken place, but not what the Catholics asserted.
Abbott, *Philomythus*, 1891, p. 193.

Eilward asked for his money, and Fulk denied [1] on oath. Then Eilward bade him pay half, as he was going to have some beer, and keep the other half for himself for beer likewise. On Fulk's still refusing, the other said he would be even with him.

"After they had both got drunk, Eilward, leaving the ale-house before the other, turned aside to Fulk's cottage, tore away the bar, burst into the house, and carried away a great grindstone and a pair of gloves, both scarcely of the value of a *nummus*. The boys, who were playing in the courtyard, cried out and, running to the tavern, called their father out to reclaim his property. Fulk followed the thief, broke the man's head with the grindstone, wounded him in the arm with a knife, brought him back to the cottage, bound him, and called in Fulk, the beadle of the village, to know what he must do with his prisoner. ' The charge,' said the beadle, ' is not heavy enough. If you tie a few more things round the prisoner and produce him thus you can accuse him of breaking the law.' The debtor agreed, and fastened round his prisoner's neck an awl, a two-edged axe, a net and some clothes, together with the grindstone and the gloves, and on the following day brought him before the king's officers.

"So, having been taken to Bedford, he was kept in the prison there for a month. He sent for a priest, in whose hearing, after confessing his sins, he vowed a pilgrimage to Jerusalem if he escaped, and he begged that he might be branded with a

[1] The debt.

cross on the shoulder. The priest branded him accordingly, but also suggested that he should seek the protection of the saints, and especially of St. Thomas, measuring his body for the length and thickness of a candle to be offered to the martyr, and also giving him a bundle of rods that self-punishment might accompany his invocations. However, the priest still sent messages to his window to comfort and strengthen him in secret. Also the Prior of Bedford often supplied him with food, visited him and had him out for a breathing-space now and then in the open air.

"At the beginning of the fifth week he was had up for trial. On his asserting that he took what he took as a pledge, and that he did not take the other articles at all, he was again remanded to prison. In the fifth week he was again tried on the charge of stealing simply the grindstone and the gloves. For the accuser, fearing to undergo the ordeal of battle demanded by the accused, condemned by silence all his previous charges, and—having on his side the viscount and the judges—managed to free himself from obligation to fight, and to secure that the accused should be tried by ordeal of water.

"Now it was the Sabbath, and the examination was put off till the third day of the following week, he himself being again kept in prison, and not allowed, by the cruelty of the keeper, vigil in the church—a right conceded by the compassion of religion to all that are to purge themselves [1] from criminal charge. In prison, however, he devoutly

---

[1] By ordeal.

kept the watch that he was not allowed to keep in the church.

"When brought out to the water-ordeal he was met by the village priest, who entreated him to bear all patiently, looking to remission of sins, to entertain no anger in his heart, to forgive all his enemies heartily, and not to despair of the compassion of God. He replied, ' May the will of God and the Martyr Thomas be fulfilled in me.'

"When plunged in the water he was found guilty. The beadle, Fulk, now seized him, saying, ' This way, rascal, this way.' ' Thanks be to God,' said the other, ' and to the holy Martyr Thomas.' Dragged to the place of execution, he was deprived of his eyes, and also mutilated according to law. As for his left eye, they at once extracted that whole; as for the right, after being lacerated and chopped to pieces, it was at last with difficulty gouged out. The members of which he had been deprived by mutilation they hid under the sod.

"He was mutilated by his accuser Fulk and the official of the same name, and also by two other executioners with them : whom, however, when they asked pardon for the love of God and St. Thomas the martyr, he freely forgave, crying aloud that he would go to the martyr's memorial, blind though he was, and persisting in the cry with a wonderful faith, knowing that it was more glorious for the martyr to restore eyes that had been taken away than to preserve them when not taken.

"He was attended now by his daughter, twelve years old, who had also begged food for him when in prison. For as all his goods were confiscated,

all his friends spurned him, and there was no one
of all those dear to him to take compassion on him.
Such a stream of blood gushed from his wounds
that in fear of his death those who were present sent
for a priest. To him he confessed. By degrees,
however, when the flow of blood was assuaged, led
by the little girl he returned to Bedford, where he
threw himself down against the wall of a house,
and all that day till evening no man showed him
kindness. But at nightfall one Eilbricht took compassion on him, and willingly welcomed him into
his house from the cold and rain.

"There, after many vigils and prayers, in the first
watch of the tenth night he whom he had invoked
appeared to Eilward in his sleep, clothed in snow-
white garments, with his pastoral staff, painting
the sign of the cross on his forehead and on his
eyeless sockets. A second time he appeared, before
dawn, bidding him persevere in watching and
praying, and place his hope in God and the Blessed
Virgin Mary and St. Thomas, who had come to
visit him : ' If, on the night of the morrow, thou
keep watch with a waxen light before the altar of
the Blessed Mary in her church close by, and devote
thyself to prayer in faith and without doubting,
thou shalt be gladdened by the restoration of thine
eyes.' The maidservant also had a similar dream.
When she told it to Eilward, he replied, ' So it may
be when it shall please God and His Blessed Martyr
Thomas.'

"When it was growing towards evening and the
sun was toward setting, the eyelids of his left eye
began to itch. In order to scratch them he removed

a waxen poultice which had been applied, either for the purpose of drawing out the purulent matter of the empty orbs or for the purpose of closing the eyelids themselves, and as by the wonderful power of God he opened his eyelids, there was seen to shine in on the house wall in front of him as it were the brightness of a lantern, for it was the red sunlight, since the sun was by this time verging toward his going down. But he, ignorant of the truth and distrusting himself about the matter, called the master of the house and showed him his fancy. ' You are mad, Eilward, you are mad,' replied his host; ' be silent, you know not what you are saying.' ' Sir,' he said, ' I assure you I am not mad, but I verily seem to myself to see as I say with my left eye.' Shaken in his mind and anxious to ascertain the truth, his host spread out his hand before his eyes, and said to him, ' Do you see that which I am doing ? ' He answered, ' Your hand is moved before my eyes and drawn this way and that.' Then he told Eilbricht in order all about his visions and the precepts or promises he had received.

"The thing was noised abroad. A multitude collected, and among them Osbern, the dean, who had control, or rather service, of the above-mentioned church. He brought the good man before the altar, instructed and strengthened his faith, and then placed a light in his hand. As soon as this was done, Eilward declared he distinctly saw the altar-cloth, then the image of the Blessed Virgin Mary, then objects of smaller size.

"The people marvelled more and more. Presently, testing the source of his sight, they detected two very small pupils latent, deep in the head, scarcely as large as the pupils of the eye of a little bird. These also incessantly increasing, prolonged by their slow augmentation the wonder of all that beheld them. The shouts of the people went up to heaven; they gave God due praise; the bells are set ringing; crowds flock in from their beds; keeping vigil with their brother who had received the gift of light, they sleeplessly await the light of the sun.

"In the morning the whole of the town gathered together, and then examining the man more closely they found that whereas before both his eyes were parti-coloured, now he had one parti-coloured but the other quite black. Now came among others the priest of St. John's Church, the same who had received Eilward's confession after mutilation. When he beheld the wonderful miracle of God, 'Why,' said he, 'do we wait for papal precept? No more delaying for me! This very moment will I begin, and conduct to the end a solemn service in the name of Thomas, the glorious friend of God, since in truth he is a martyr beyond price. Who can hesitate to give the name of martyr to one who does such mighty and such merciful deeds?' So he ran to his church, set the bells ringing, and was as good as his word.

"Now no longer bereft of light, but bedecked therewith, even as he had been dragged with ignominy through the midst of the town to endure his punishment, so now through the self-same street amid the praise and applause of the people he was led back to the Church of St. Paul, where also he passed the eve of the Lord's Day in vigil. Departing thence, he hastened his journey to St. Thomas, the author of his restoration. Whatever gifts folk gave him, he bestowed on the poor for love of the martyr. . . . On his coming to London he was received by Hugh, Bishop of Durham, who would not let him go from himself till he had sent a messenger to Bedford and had been certified of the facts after diligent inquiry.

"But even after we had received him in our house at Canterbury, although he had been preceded by the testimony of very many witnesses, yet we did not feel satisfied till we heard the substance of the above-written statements confirmed by the letter and testimony of the citizens of Bedford. For they directed to us a document of which the contents were as follows—

"' The Burgesses of Bedford to the Convent of Canterbury and to all the faithful in Christ, health ! Be it known to the Convent of Canterbury and, further, to all Catholics, that God hath wrought in Bedford a wonderful and illustrious miracle on account of the merits of the most holy Thomas the martyr. For it happened that a countryman of Westoning, Eilward by name, for some theft of the value of only one *nummus*, having been taken and brought before the viscount of Bedford and before the knights of the county, and having been by them publicly condemned, was deprived of his eyes and privy members in the presence of clergy and laity, men and women. This is also testified by the chaplain of St. John in Bedford, to whom the aforesaid countryman confessed.[1] And this same is testified by his host, Eilbricht by name, in whose house he was afterwards received—namely, that he was entirely without eyes and testicles when first he was received in his house. And afterwards invoking oftentimes the merits of St. Thomas the Martyr, by an apparition of the aforesaid martyr, he was gloriously and wonderfully restored to health.'"[2]

William, a monk of Canterbury, relates a similar mutilation and a similar miraculous healing by St. Thomas, which took place at Durham, testified to by Hugh de Puiset, Bishop of Durham, and Benedict gives a third which happened at Corbie, testified by a letter to the Convent of Canterbury from the Prior and Convent of Corbie.[3]

Other works of healing wrought by St. Thomas include, beside the cure of blindness, complaint in the head, swelling in the arm, paralysis, disease of the liver, danger in child-bearing, fever, tumour, dumbness, lameness, gout and madness. Miracles of healing began so soon after the martyrdom as the third day (in the case of Emma, wife of a Sussex knight, who, while weeping for Thomas as a martyr, recovered from a temporary blindness), and so soon as the fifth day in so distant a part of the country as Gloucestershire, where Huelina recovered from a long-standing complaint in the head, immediately after Aalisa, her mother, had in London confessed her faith in Thomas as a martyr

---

[1] After mutilation.
[2] E. A. Abbott, *St. Thomas of Canterbury*, 1898, 2 vols. vol. ii. 80 ff.
[3] *Ibid.*, ii. 103 ff.

and pledged her daughter to go on pilgrimage to the place of death. This last, therefore, is a case of "absent treatment." Miracles were wrought not only on visitors to the tomb of the martyr, but on those who were aspersed by the "Water of Canterbury," or were touched by a handkerchief which the archbishop had blessed. On the other hand, many pilgrims to Canterbury went back without being cured, and in the case of two boys the martyr himself announced that he would not do anything for them. Benedict himself describes the diversities of cure in respect of time, "how some received it at the time of their vow; others on the way to Canterbury, but a long way off; others on coming into the city; others in the cathedral or at the tomb. Some were healed in the moment of departure; some not till they had returned to their homes." [1]

St. Ubaldo

The cult of this saint affords so excellent an example of the belief which is a necessary condition of spiritual healing, that our survey of mediæval healing may well include a brief account of it. Ubaldo was born in Gubbio, an ancient town situated on the western slope of Monte Ingino in the Central Apennines. Dedicated to the religious life, he became prior of the cathedral, then Bishop-elect of Perugia, and finally bishop in his own native city. A life of holiness resulted in the work-

[1] E. A. Abbott, *St. Thomas of Canterbury*, i. 286.

ing of miracles. His prayers restored to health a dying monk; his touch cured blindness; a paralysed woman who seized his vestment when he was consecrating a church was immediately healed. Another blind man sent to the bishop by an injunction given in a dream recovered his sight, and a priest was cured of a swollen hand. Ubaldo died on May 15, 1160, and that day has been a feast-day at Gubbio down to the present time.

As is usual, the death of the saint was the occasion of an augmentation of his miraculous powers. The first to be healed was a paralytic woman who touched the corpse. "This miracle was followed by a succession of others. During the four days he remained unburied he caused the blind to see, the deaf to hear, the lame to walk. He performed many other miracles, and is said to have dispensed health to the sick of all sorts, as if he were some physician sent from heaven."

Again, another increase of power sets in after burial. "The first wonders narrated of the saint, when laid to his holy rest, are compared to the acts of a prince entering into his kingdom. He at once cast out multitudinous demons and expelled all sorts of diseases and infirmities. The names of several persons are given who were relieved of evil spirits. . . . A considerable list is also furnished [1] of marvellous cures performed by the dead saint. An appendix based on a different manuscript (pars 31–34), ascribes to God and to St. Ubaldo liberation from captivity and shipwreck, as well as healings." Pilgrimages were made to his shrine from all parts

[1] In the *Acta Sanctorum*, May 16.

of Italy, as they were made to Epidauros before the Christian era, and as they are made to Treves and Lourdes to-day. Water was blessed and used in healing. Oil was taken from the lamp burning before the sacred corpse and similarly used. The expulsion of demons from the bodies of persons possessed by them might be almost regarded as the saint's speciality. From one person he expelled 2,999 out of 3,000 demons, leaving one as a sort of thorn in the flesh to discipline the patient and increase her virtue. From another he drove out as many as 13,000, and from a third he expelled as many as 400,000 in four days.

If the use of water and oil reminds us of the "Water of Canterbury" and of the oil taken from wonder-working shrines, the miracles of deliverance from perils remind us of the similar wonders ascribed to Cosmas and Damian, and so take us back to the Dioscuri. These latter, indeed, are all of the same type and rest on an invocation of the saint made in mortal peril. Thus a tree he was felling came down on Agnello Brugnori, but did not hurt him because he invoked in time St. Ubaldo. Giovanni Marcello, a furrier, on being carried away by a torrent, was saved by an old man, who pulled him out by his hair on his invoking the saint. A child fell into boiling water and was pulled out unhurt, thanks again to Ubaldo. A soldier wounded in battle could not pull out the iron from the wound. The saint, however, did it for him, exactly as we read Asklepios had done before him. A woman, Simonia of Gubbio, fell into a well and was saved from being drowned because Our Lady and Ubaldo held up her chin until she could be pulled up. Moreover, the saint protected his native city and also other cities from their enemies. He punished his traducers even with death. "He released prisoners, assisted births and allayed other discomforts." In Mr. Bower's words, "if we examine the catalogue, we shall find Ubaldo to have been, and perhaps still to be, reputed not merely as the nominal patron of Gubbio, but as a miracle-worker upon the hill, at the stream, a protector and healer of the people, a saviour of the State, powerful over flocks and weather, a terror to foes of Gubbio and to all evil spirits." [1]

But for our present purpose the interesting point in the above legends of miracles is not so much the question how far they may be treated as history, nor even the testimony they bear to the psychology of the people who, at all events, believed in them and perhaps invented some of them. For a far more interesting question lies in the background, viz. as to the relation of these Christian miracles to the similar miracles of which undoubted, if all too scanty, records have come down to us. The continuity of history, like the continuity of nature, is a commonplace of modern culture, and miracles, in the strict sense of arbitrary acts breaking into the continuum, receive no favour from science. Hence a belief in Ubaldo's "miracles" presupposes a similar belief in earlier "miracles." And the

[1] See *Acta Sanctorum*, May 16, vol. xvi. pp. 625–636, and the admirable monograph of Mr. Herbert M. Bower on *The Elevation and Procession of the Ceri at Gubbio*, published for the Folk-Lore Society in 1897, from which the quotations in the above account are taken.

transition from the pagan to the Christian was made all the easier by the probably wise decision of Christian authority at the turning-point to accept pagan customs and to change their names when adopting them. Thus Gregory, writing to the Abbot Mellitus about Augustine's mission, counselled that "very little destruction of idols' temples should be made among the people. But let the idols themselves that are in them be destroyed, water blessed and sprinkled in those temples, altars constructed and relics deposited. . . . And since it is the habit to kill many oxen in sacrifice to demons, therefore as to these also some alteration of observance ought to be made, so that the people may for themselves make booths from branches of trees about those churches which are changed from the temples, and may observe a solemnity with religious feasts on the day of dedication or birth of the holy martyrs whose relics are there deposited." [1]

Similarly, Gregory Thaumaturgus, "on account of the pleasures they enjoyed at pagan festivals, granted to the country-folk leave to pursue enjoyments in celebrating the memory of holy martyrs," and this conduct was explicitly approved of by Gregory of Nyssa in his encomium of his predecessor. And Augustine of Hippo, writing to Alypius of Tagaste, describes the difficulty he met with in his attempts to check inordinate banqueting in the church itself in honour of the martyrs. He goes on to say that he was twitted with going counter to his predecessors who had allowed those

[1] The letter is given in Bede, *H. E.*, i. 30, Plummer's ed. vol. i. p. 65.

banquets, and he replies that they did so because of the crowds of heathen who brought into the church their festival customs, and could not be at once and wholly deprived of them. "Therefore it seemed good to our ancestors that this weakness should be gently dealt with, and that the festival days should be celebrated after those which they were abandoning, in honour of the holy martyrs, if not with similar sacrilege, at least with similar delights."[1] Augustine, though he disliked the excesses indulged in, had no other objection apparently to the custom, and is, at all events, a good witness to the antiquity of the ecclesiastical diplomacy which knew how to bridge over the old and the new.

The difficulty of tracing the links which bind the earlier religion to its supplanter, prompted Plutarch's *Romane Questions*, in which he propounds a series of questions such as the science of Folk-lore is in the habit of asking. That his answers are insufficient is easily accountable for by the lack of the comparative study of religion then existing. But Plutarch bears ample evidence to our contention that history is a continuum, and that the chief difference between Paganism and Christianity is that the one came before the other. As Dr. F. B. Jevons says: "No form of religion is easily or at once rooted out, even by a new religion. A *modus vivendi* has to be found between the old faith and the new. The animal, which was once itself worshipped, is tolerated merely as the symbol of some divine attribute. The nixies con-

[1] Ep. XXIX. in Benedict. ed. ii. 52.

tinue to ply their old calling under the new name of Old Nick." [1]

So Grimm says: "The result of a new religion coming in is mixture with the old, which never dies out entirely. The old faith then becomes a superstition." [2]

It is worth noticing, as illustrating the way in which a blend of old and new came about, that St. Augustine's remark as to the memorials of the martyrs taking place on the day after the pagan festival (dies festos post eos quos relinquebant) receives unexpected corroboration from the fact that St. Ubaldo's day in the Roman Calendar is May 16, while the feast-day at Gubbio is May 15. Further, the Gubbio ceremonies are distinctly of a pagan and not a Christian character. From this we may infer that Gubbio still, in fact without knowing it, commemorates not the great spiritual healer, Ubaldo, but Mercury, whose birthday was kept in Rome on May 15. But Mercury in Italy attracted to his cult that of Evander or Pan; he was the god of good-fortune, of success in commerce, the protecting god of States, and his cult was found in Præneste before it existed in Rome. Moreover, his cult was established in all parts of Italy, in Campania, Etruria, Apulia, Lucania and Sicily among others. The conjecture, therefore, is not too hazardous that Gubbio to-day honours on May 15 Mercurius Euphrosynus, under the name of St. Ubaldo the Spiritual Healer and Wonder-worker of the twelfth century. Again, we see that the

---

[1] Plutarch's *Romane Questions*, 1892, p. xlvi.
[2] *Teut. Mythol.*, iv. 1699.

G

division between Paganism and Catholicism is
more diagrammatic than real. Spiritual Healing
flourishes under the one in the same way as under
the other.[1]

ST. MARTIN OF TOURS

The late Dean Farrar [2] says roundly: "Most, if
not all, of the so-called miracles which were supposed to surround Martin with a blaze of glory
were either absolutely and on the face of them
false; or were gross exaggerations of natural events;
or were subjective impressions clothed in objective
images; or were the distortions of credulous
rumour; or at the best cannot claim in their favour
a single particle of trustworthy evidence. They
cannot be related as though they were actual events.
Martin was an eminent bishop, but half of the
wonderful deeds attributed to him are unworthy and
absurd." It would not be difficult to picture a critic
whose mental attitude to the New Testament was
that of Dean Farrar to ecclesiastical miracles saying exactly the same thing of the New Testament.
On the other hand, Sulpicius Severus, to whom we
are chiefly indebted for what we know of St. Martin,
says: "I implore those who are to read what follows
to give full faith to the things narrated, and to
believe that I have written nothing of which I had

[1] W. H. Roscher, *Ausführliches Lexicon*, s. v. *Hermes*. It
is just possible that the St. George and St. Antony who are
associated with St. Ubaldo as inferior to him at Gubbio, may
represent an earlier Castor and Pollux, who in their turn gave
way to a Hermes as he later did to Ubaldo.
[2] *Lives of the Fathers*, i. 644.

not certain knowledge and evidence." And in his *Dialogues* he introduces a "Gallic friend," a disciple of Martin, prefacing an account of his master's miracles with the assertion : "I shall relate nothing which I simply heard from others, but only events of which I myself was an eye-witness." [1]

Among the acts of Spiritual Healing which he then proceeds to relate are the following : (1) A boy bitten by a poisonous serpent, all but lifeless and with his whole body swollen, was placed at Martin's feet. The saint put his finger to the bitten place, when the poison was drawn thither from all parts of the body and came out mixed with blood, "just as milk flows from the teats of goats or sheep when these are squeezed by the hands of shepherds. The boy rose up quite well."

(2) Before he was bishop he restored two dead men to life, but while he was bishop he raised up only one. This last took place in a heathen village, a woman of which brought with outstretched hands the lifeless body of her son to the blessed man, saying : "We know that you are a friend of God : restore me my son, who is my only one." The saint, perceiving that he could manifest power, kneeled by the body in prayer, and then, rising, delivered the boy to his mother. Then the whole multitude acknowledged Christ as God.

(3) Martin's power of exorcism was great. "He touched no one with his hands and reproached no one in words . . . but the possessed being brought up to him he ordered all others to depart; and the doors being bolted, clothed in sackcloth and

[1] *Dial.*, i. Chap. XXVII.

sprinkled with ashes, he stretched himself on the ground in the midst of the church and turned to prayer. Then truly might one behold the wretched beings (*i. e.* the demons) tortured with various results, some hanging as it were from a cloud with their feet turned upwards . . . while in another part of the church one could see them tortured without any question being addressed to them and confessing their crimes."[1] The Gaul says later:[2] "I saw afterwards a person possessed brought to him at the gate of the monastery, and that before the man touched the threshold he was cured."

In the *Life* Severus relates the following: (1) A certain girl at Treves was so completely prostrated by a terrible paralysis that for a long time she had been quite unable to make use of her body for any purpose, and being as it were already dead, only the smallest breath of life seemed still to remain in her. When Martin came to Treves and entered the church, a multitude being there and many bishops, the father embraced the saint's knees and besought him to visit his daughter and heal her. The saint was bewildered and shrank from the task, saying it was not in his hands, but finally he consented and went. There he first of all prayed, then asked for oil and poured some into her mouth, whereupon first her voice returned, and then, through contact with him, her limbs began one by one to recover life, till at last, in the presence of the people, she arose with firm steps.[3]

---

[1] *Dial.*, ii. 6.   [2] *Ibid.*, ii. 14.
[3] *Life*, Chap. XVI.

(2) In Chapter XIX Severus throws together a few examples, as he says, out of a multitude, lest his readers should find him tedious. The daughter of Arborius, an ex-prefect, was cured from the burning fever of a quartan ague merely by a letter which her father had received from the saint. A man named Paulinus suffering from cataract—having a nubes, cloud or "pretty thick skin" nearly covering up the pupil of his eye—was cured by Martin touching his eye with a painter's brush. The saint himself having fallen downstairs, and being tortured with grievous sufferings and lying at the point of death, was cured instantaneously by an angel, who came to him in his cell and washed his wounds. Martin once, when entering Paris, gave a kiss to a leper, who was at once cured from all his misery, and gave thanks in the church the next day with a healthy skin. It is also affirmed that threads from the garment of the blessed man or from his sackcloth cured many that were sick, for by either being tied round the fingers or placed about the neck, they very often drove away diseases from the afflicted.

(3) The two miracles of restoring a dead man to life are given.[1] The first was a catechumen, who suddenly died of a fever before being baptized. Martin went to the cell where the body was lying, stretched himself on it, prayed, and then, perceiving that power was present (*adesse virtutem*), he waited patiently for the issue. After two hours the dead man began to move a little in all his members, and to tremble with his eyes open for the practice of

[1] *Life*, Chaps. VII. and VIII.

sight. Afterwards he related how, when his spirit
was led for judgment he received a severe sentence,
and that when two angels suggested he was the man
for whom Martin was praying, the order was given
that he should be given up to Martin, and so he
was restored to life. The second case was that of
one of the slaves of Lupicinus, whom Martin
restored to life by the same methods after the slave
had hanged himself.

Analogy would lead us to expect that St. Martin's
relics would be even more efficacious against sickness than the living saint had been, and St. Gregory
of Tours assures us that they were. Out of seven
books he wrote on Miracles, he devotes four to those
worked by the relics of St. Martin. A man in
Italy, suffering from a tumour, begged for a piece
of the garment of a man who had visited the saint's
tomb, and this, being placed on the tumour, banished
it. The saint appeared to a certain abbess in a
dream and told her he was prevented from returning
to Gaul because of a sick man, a certain Placidus,
who was lying at her gate sick. When the abbess
arose and told her vision to the sick man, he had
sufficient faith to recover from his desperate sickness.[1] A woman named Bella, whose sight was
gone, insisted that, if taken to Martin's tomb, the
saint who had cured a leper with a kiss would also
cure her, which duly came to pass.[2] A man tongue-
tied and with paralysed hand, was cured by the
saint, but when his master put him again to
work his malady returned, and was only again
removed by his return to the saint's remains.[3] St.

[1] *De Miraculis*, i. 16.   [2] *Ibid.*, i. 19.   [3] *Ibid.*, i. 22.

Gregory says that he knew himself a woman emaciated by five months' dysentery who was cured by drinking some of the dust of the blessed tomb, and then walked back home instead of being carried.[1]

Similarly, blind, paralysed, dumb, feverish, possessed and similarly afflicted persons were in great numbers cured, and the accounts of their being so cured fill the whole of the second and third books of *De Miraculis*. But as they are all alike in their misery and in their cure, there is no need to recount them. A visit to the shrine, or the application of water with which the saint's dust had been mixed, or of oil from his altar, was frequently enough to gain the boon of health. The feast of the saint, November 11, was especially a day notable for the cures effected.[2]

One or two remarks may be made on the general character of these mediæval stories of Spiritual Healing.

(*a*) They are signalized by an entire absence of the critical spirit, or of any sense of "values." Wonders worked by a saint are all equally useful as proof of special miraculous powers as still residing in the Catholic Church.

(*b*) Some allowance, therefore, must be made for the bias of ecclesiastical interest in the same way

---

[1] *De Miraculis*, i. 37.

[2] Alban Butler, *Lives of the Primitive Fathers, Martyrs, and other Principal Saints*, 1799, vol. xi, under November 15 ; S. Baring-Gould, *Lives of the Saints*, 2nd ed., 1877, November 11 ; Sulpicii Severi, *Libri qui supersunt*, Ed. Halm, Vienna, 1876 ; *Nicene and Post-Nicene Fathers*, ed. Wace and Schaff, vol. xi. 1894, pp. 3–54 ; Gregorius Turon, in Migne, vol. lxxi. col. 913–1010.

that we must allow for it when interpreting the inscriptions in the Abaton at Epidauros.

(c) We can hardly describe the wonders wrought by saints in the Middle Age as "miracles," for a miracle presupposes a fixed law of Nature, and of such a law the ecclesiastical world of that age had no conception.

(d) The healing wonders, in common with other wonders related, are based to a large extent on the Gospel wonders and reproduce them. It is not, therefore, an unreasonable suspicion that the same feeling may have been at work in those who recorded the Gospel works of healing. Certainly the formulæ in the later stories are an imitation of the formulæ used in the earlier.

(e) In the later stories, however, there is less restraint and an absence of the sense of "value" which the New Testament on the whole does reveal. In the Middle Age, for example, it is all one with the pious scribe whether the disease removed is "organic" or "functional." A powerful saint may as well make a new eye-ball as remove a contraction of a muscle. St. John Damascene, for example, among others tells of the Jewish priest who contemptuously pushed the bier on which the body of the Virgin Mary was being conveyed to the grave, and whose hands were instantly severed from the arm at the wrist. St. Peter, however, bade him put his stumps near the severed hands, when they grew together again.

(f) The relics of the saint, or anything which he had touched, were as efficacious for healing as the living saint himself. This witnesses to two things :

(1) the fact that wonder-working generally and Spiritual Healing in particular were in the air, and were accepted as part of the work which the Church was there to do; and (2) that the general belief of the age did not regard death as setting up the barrier between this life and the next, which Protestantism has taught us to regard as rigid.

(g) Finally, when every possible allowance is made for fraud, credulity, exaggeration, interested motives and the love of the marvellous, it is probable that there remains a residuum of fact around which the glowing shrine has been builded. It is not likely that the belief in wonders would have persisted for more than 1,200 years unless it had been fed from time to time by some supplies of fact, however small the supply may have been. And when we come to modern times, times, that is, whose records we can sift, judge and control, we shall be in a position to determine with some precision what the nature of that fact was.

*   *   *

As a foil to these wonder-works we may glance for a moment at the mixed medical and Spiritual Healing which obtained in an infirmary under "religious" in the thirteenth century. The infirmary of a cell of Friars Preachers at that period was a building by itself apart with its own self-contained suite of apartments, and a garden in which the convalescent might walk. The head of it was a Friar in whom were found an immovable patience and ready sympathy. He might be himself trained in the medical art, but in any case his duty was to see that the sick had every material and spiritual care. He was to have the tenderness of a mother, remembering that the Scripture says : [1] "The sick man groans where there is no woman" to nurse him. In the infirmary were treated not only outsiders but the Friars themselves when they were sick by the important personage, who was at once barber, surgeon, physician and dentist. His surgical methods were so excruciatingly painful that it was lamentable to hear the patient cry as a woman in child-birth while the cutting away of his flesh was going on.

When a Friar's death-hour seemed near all was done to add spiritual consolation to material help. The Office was recited, a dry or white Mass was celebrated ; at the first symptoms of the death-agony a Friar summoned the community by beating on a wooden gong, and they would run to the sick-room saying their Credo ; the dying man was placed on a bed of ashes, while around him his brethren recited the Litanies of the saints, the Penitential Psalms, to which was afterwards added the *Salve Regina*. Nothing mournful was said or done; these men died with joy of their God.[2] The pious Dominican gives a prose which was found in a Dominican Processional of the thirteenth century belonging to an unknown convent; it was composed for the purpose of comforting the sick and of turning their

[1] Ecclus. xxxvi. 25, "ubi non est mulier ingemiscit aeger" ; rather the meaning is that a man without a good wife is a wanderer and homeless.

[2] R. P. Mortier, *Histoire des Maîtres Généraux de l'ordre des Frères Prêcheurs*, A.D. 1170-1263, tome i, p. 592 ff.

thoughts to God. As an instrument of Spiritual Healing it deserves a place here.

1
O dulcis Frater, si recedis,
Cor tuum non doleat,
Sed quod placere Deo credis
Hoc et tibi placeat.

2
Quis dolet si pericula
Maris evadit citius?
Quis evadens in tabula
Vult esse portu longius?

3
Fratres cuncti qui sunt
Juncti beato Dominico
Cum videbunt te gaudebunt
Et occurrent ilico.

4
Exultabunt quod liberatus
De tanto naufragio
Eorum sis associatus
Felici collegio.

5
Ordinis observatio
Te ducet ad hunc exitum,
Et pia Christi passio
Quæ vincit omne meritum.

6
Certus esto quod sint præsto
Angelici spiritus
Ut te portent et confortent
Hora tui transitus.

7
Nec tibi Mater pietatis
Sua claudet viscera,
Sed tuis orans pro peccatis
Aderit opifera.

8
Tunc tuas terget lacrymas,
Benigna Dei dextera,
Et inter sanctas animas
Loca dabit florigera.

9
Ubi vernos et æternos
Flores admiraberis,
Ubi sine quovis fine
Felix spatiaberis.

10
Quanta tibi Deus ibi
Bona præparaverit
Meditari sive fari
Nullus vivens poterit.

11
Ergo cum tu sis intraturus
In Domini gaudium
Curre jam lætus et securus
Ad supernum bravium.

12
Nec cures de scientia ;
Nec si dimittis studium,
Nam cito scies omnia
In causa studens omnium.

13
Ad Dei forte gloriam
Sperabas magna facere ;
Sed ejus providentiam
Non oportet instruere.

14
Jesus qui novit plenius
Quid electis expediat,
De te quod est utilius
Tibi clementer faciat.   Amen.

CHAPTER V

SPIRITUAL HEALING IN MODERN TIMES

SPIRITUAL HEALING, though by no means extinguished by the scepticism which began its salutary work from the fifteenth century onwards, was unquestionably deprived of its vogue. The atmosphere was no longer charged with credulity; relics were roundly described as "pigges bones," and thaumaturgic saints denounced as impostors. Yet Martin Luther is said to have performed cures. The Moravians and Waldenses trusted to prayer and anointing, as the Peculiar People do to-day. These latter were founded by John Banyard in London in 1838, and they order their dealings with sickness strictly on the provisions of Jas. v. 14. The Mormons, too, believe in faith-healing, and Joseph Smith's instructions to them are to "trust in God when sick, and live by faith and not by medicine or poison." They hold to the gifts of prophecy, miracles and the casting out of devils. The Society of Friends in England and Pietism in Germany, as well as the Methodism of the eighteenth century, have sporadic examples of Spiritual Healing which show that the force from which it springs, though less generally active, was by no means extinct. In fact the phenomena of this period, though seemingly barren of result in this field, yet serve the useful purpose of pointing us to the real character of Spiritual Healing. They show us clearly that the power correlated with "faith" will produce the gifts of healing when it is generally and implicitly believed in, and that with the lessening of the intensity of faith goes automatically a restriction of those gifts. In the Middle Age Spiritual Healing was common because everybody believed in it and expected it. Hence the supply met the demand. But after the Reformation people began to question it, as they began to question all things, and accordingly the demand being less the supply sank proportionately. There is, therefore, a close and a necessary connection established by Nature between Faith and Spiritual Healing.

It will be enough to take two men as representing the activity of Spiritual Healing in the days immediately preceding our own, Valentine Greatrakes the Stroker and Prince Hohenlohe-Waldenburg-Schillingsfürst.

Valentine Greatrakes[1] "the Stroker" is an example from the seventeenth century of the method of healing with which we are concerned. Born in the County of Waterford on February 14, 1628–9, and educated in England, he became convinced in 1662 that he had the power of curing the King's evil. On being put to the test his power was proved, and the next four years were largely spent in curing or in trying to cure people of scrofula, ague, rheumatism and similar ailments, first in Ireland and then for a year in England. He met with varying success, and no rational ex-

[1] *Dictionary of National Biography*, 1890, vol. xxiii.

planation has been given either by himself or others of his failures. His method was the laying on of his hand with the prayer: "God Almighty heal thee for His mercy's sake." He did not himself regard his power as miraculous, but said that "he had reason to believe that there was something in it of an extraordinary gift of God." From 1666 till his death in 1683 he treated patients occasionally only.

In the last century the most striking figure in the annals of spiritual healing is that of Prince Hohenlohe - Waldenburg - Schillingsfürst, born August 17, 1794, educated at Vienna, Tyrnan, and in the Catholic University of Ellwangen, ordained priest in 1815, made a canon of Grandwaradin (or Grosswardein), and ending his life on November 14, 1849. Nothing would have raised him out of the common order of exemplary priests had he not chanced to become acquainted in 1821 with the curé of Harfort and his brother-in-law, a simple peasant named Martin-Michel. This latter had an unbounded faith in the power of prayer, and on one occasion when the Prince was to preach the next day a sermon on the Feast of the Purification of the Blessed Virgin Mary, and was suffering from an intense pain in the neck, Martin and he kneeled down in prayer, and the trouble immediately disappeared.

Soon after the Prince discovered that he himself could become a curative agent, and as his own description of the discovery puts him in a vivid light before us it may be quoted at length.

"When we sat down to dinner," he says, "the

servants brought in the young Princess, Matilda von Schwarzenberg, who, through paralysis, had lost for eight years the power of walking. She was placed near me. Touched with compassion for her, and thinking of my good Martin-Michel, I said to myself : ' If that man was able to obtain healing for my violent malady, he might perhaps do the same for this child, if she has a firm trust in the help of the Lord.' I was careful, however, not to say anything about my feelings to anybody, knowing too well how the world would ridicule me. After dinner I went for a walk in the town, and not being able to get away from my thoughts I made up my mind that if the thing was to be, God would determine its mode. It was on June 19, 1821. The evening of the same day, after having said my breviary and, if I may say so, being very piously disposed, I spent the whole evening with the curé and Martin-Michel, without mentioning, however, the invalid. On the 21st, while offering the holy sacrifice of the Mass, I felt myself, after the consecration, strongly moved, and impelled to go to the Princess's to tell her that she would be helped by Jesus Christ, if she had a firm belief in his words : ' Verily, verily I say unto you, whatsoever ye shall ask the Father in my name He will give it you.' It was impossible for me to get rid of the thought during the rest of the holy sacrifice. When I got into the sacristy I turned on myself, and after reflection I tried to banish from my mind the idea as springing from a lively imagination. All my efforts, however, were in vain. I felt myself all the more impelled to go to visit the Princess, accom-

panied by Martin-Michel. I went, and bade my
companion wait in the ante-chamber, going alone
into the chamber of the Princess, to whom I said
without any preamble : ' My dear cousin, God can
help you by Jesus Christ, His Son.' ' Yes,' she
replied, ' without doubt; that is what I believe.'
I then went on : ' I have brought with me a pious
peasant by whose prayers God has already helped
some sick folk. If you will allow me, I will go
and fetch him, that he may pray for you.' ' With
all my heart,' she replied. Martin-Michel then
came in, and the following conversation took place :
' Is not God, your Highness, Almighty ?—that is
why He can help us. And being infinitely good
He wills also to help us. He is truly our Father ;
ought not that thought to kindle our hope ? We
ought to have a firm trust in Him through Jesus
Christ, who said : "If ye ask anything in my name
He will give it you." None the less our prayer
should begin and end : "what God wills," or, "as
God wills," or "because God wills." ' After these
words, the good peasant joined his hands in prayer.
One must have seen him to form an idea of the
recollection and the fervour with which he prayed.
The prayer finished, I cannot tell how it was, but
I felt a secret power which commanded me to cry
aloud to the Princess : '' In the name of Jesus
Christ, rise up and walk.' When I had uttered
these words, for me so memorable, the Princess
was set free from her bonds, and was able not only
to stand on her feet, a thing she had not done for
eight years, but was also able to walk. My tears
flowed, and I could say nothing but ' My God, my

God! is it possible?' As soon as the news of this wonderful event was spread abroad I found myself surrounded by sick people, but in fact I hardly knew what took place at the time. Also, I will say nothing about many things which took place then and afterwards, because about them it is not for me to judge. I am a son of the Church, and will be always faithful to her. Let Rome decide after my death whether my life was in accordance with my faith. But I know that in life there are moments and hours of holy rapture when the soul is absorbed in God." [1]

From this time onwards the Prince was sought after by crowds who needed his help. He and Martin-Michel prayed together for them, and were careful to tell them the hour of these prayers, so that the sick might pray also at the same time. The Court of Rome does not appear to have been unsympathetic to the Prince on the whole, and the Pope sent him his apostolic benediction. For the next twenty-six years the Prince exercised in peace his double rôle of a Catholic priest and spiritual healer, until in 1849 he was obliged through dropsy, the illness which proved afterwards fatal, to give up his work and retire to Grosswardein. He died, however, on the way thither, after having treated, it is said, in the last twelve months of his life no fewer than 18,000 people. He does not seem to have practised the laying on of hands, but trusted entirely to prayer for his cures, and he left behind him a small body of prayers and devotions.

[1] *Biographie Universelle* (Michaud) *Ancienne et Moderne*, 1857, vol. 19, s. v. Cf. *Nouvelle Biographie Générale*, Paris, 1858, vol. 24.

The Prince, however, was but continuing a tradition of which John Joseph Gassner,[1] a Roman Catholic priest in Swabia, was a representative about the middle of the eighteenth century. Gassner differed from the Prince in the point that he attributed all sickness to demoniacal possession, and regarded his own work as that of exorcism. His methods were not unlike those of Mesmer,[2] whom he met in Switzerland and influenced so far that Mesmer, through his example, abandoned the use of magnets as curative instruments.

Reference has already been made to Martin Luther, and it is recorded of him that he on one occasion found Melancthon lying dangerously ill at Weimar. After praying with him he took him by the hand, and exclaimed: "Be of good cheer, Philip, thou wilt not die. . . . Give not place to the spirit of grief, nor become the slayer of thyself, but trust in the Lord." Melancthon recovered, and Luther afterwards testified: "I found him dead, but by an evident miracle of God he lives." To his friend Myconius, who was dying from consumption, Luther wrote: "May God not let me hear so long as I live that you are dead, but cause you to survive me. I pray this earnestly, and will have it granted and my will shall be done herein, Amen." Myconius was so horrified by this blasphemy that he recovered.

So Bullinger testified to cures being effected among his people. "Through confidence in the

[1] *Allgemeine Deutsche Biographie*, Leipzig, 1878, band 8, p. 407.
[2] *Op. cit.*, band xxi. p. 487.

name of Christ, members greatly afflicted and shattered with disease are restored afresh to health."

Richard Baxter declared that he had known the prayer of faith to save the sick when all physicians had given them up as dead, and he testifies that he had himself been relieved of a hard tumour on one of his tonsils by his preaching about his past deliverances.

George Fox records in his journals a number of cures of which he had been an eye-witness, and refers particularly to insanity, scrofula and epilepsy as among them.

Count Zinzendorf told John Wesley that among his Moravians apostolic powers had showed themselves "in the healing of maladies in themselves incurable, such as cancers and consumptions, when the patient was in the agonies of death, all by means of prayer, or of a single word." Wesley himself afterwards was, he tells us, cured of fever and great pain by calling on Jesus Christ, and on another occasion he was relieved of weariness and headache and his horse of lameness, both at the same time. He also refers in his *Journal* to cases of rupture, tumours and prolapsus uteri being cured among Methodists.

The Mormons claim that cases of cancer, consumption and small-pox have been cured among them without the use of medicines, and one of their apostles declared that "he alone in the good old days of faith in 1849 and 1850 performed more and more wonderful cures than Christ Himself, raising the dead only excepted."

Father Mathew, the famous temperance advocate,

is another witness, and almost against his will. Among the cures effected by his prayers and blessings were cases of partial blindness, lameness, insanity and hysteria. Even so late as the middle of the last century Dorothea Trüdel, a flower-worker of the Swiss village of Männedorf, became famous for the cures she effected in answer to prayer. She was tried before the court in consequence and in the course of the trial testimony was given to hundreds of cases of healing. Her work was continued after her death by a M. Zeller.

Pastor Blumhardt is another example of a man who, believing on the name of Jesus, put his belief to the proof in the case of sickness, and became famous for the cures wrought through him. Pastor Rein of South Germany is another Spiritual Healer, and Pastor Stockmayer of Hauptwiel in Switzerland another.

The best-known body of Faith Healers in England have their head-quarters at Bethshan House in the north of London, and branches in many of the provincial towns, and in the colonies. At the International Faith-healing Conference held in London in 1885 some 200 or 300 persons testified that they had been healed by faith, and in Australia 1,100 were found to give the same testimony. Almost every disease figures in their list of cures.

The "Peculiar People" also trust to prayer when they are ill, and refuse to see a doctor even for broken bones. And at Salvation Army meetings, according to Major Pearson, prayer has been found effectual against disease.

There is no need to do more than place on record the admirably sane and very successful work done by the Rev. Dr. Worcester, the Rev. Dr. McComb, and Dr. Coriat at Emmanuel Church, Boston, U.S.A., which has been deliberately limited to cases of so-called functional disorder. No similar movement has yet been inaugurated on the same scale, or with the same equipment under the auspices of any Christian body in the United Kingdom.

Professor E. B. Tylor quotes a case of a miraculous cure which took place in Rome in 1870.[1] According to this story "an Italian lady, afflicted with a tumour and incipient cancer, was exhorted by a Jesuit priest to recommend herself to the Blessed John Berchmans, a pious Jesuit novice from Belgium, who died in 1621 and was beatified in 1865. Her adviser procured for her ' three small packets of dust gathered from the coffin of this saintly innocent, a little cross made of the boards of the room the blessed youth occupied, as well as some portion of the wadding in which his venerable head was wrapped.' During nine days' devotion the patient accordingly invoked the Blessed John, swallowed small portions of his dust in water, and at last pressed the cross to her breast so vehemently that she was seized with sickness, went to sleep, and awoke without a symptom of the complaint. And when Dr. Panegrossi, the physician, beheld the incredible cure, and heard that the patient had

---

[1] *Primitive Culture*, 4th ed. 11, 122, quoting "A New Miracle at Rome, being an Account of a Miraculous Cure," London, (Washbourne), 1870.

addressed herself to the Blessed Berchmans, he bowed his head, saying, ' When such physicians interfere *we* have nothing more to say.' " It is obvious that there is no need to assume here any miraculous exercise of power by the Blessed Berchmans. The belief of the priest aided by the use of venerated relics acting on a susceptible nature, and one moreover at the time excited by a strong desire for health, is quite sufficient to set going a process in which the life-force in the patient was stimulated to such activity as to clear away the obstruction to its freedom. Here, as generally in similar cases, the *vera causa* may be found within the limits of Nature, if only Nature be not separated from God, but seen to be the organ through which He works. "The help that is done upon earth He doeth it Himself."

LOURDES

The way in which the "miracles" at Lourdes should be treated [1] can hardly be better exemplified than by a sympathetic though impartial writer in the *Spectator* of September 3, 1898, who will bear a lengthy quotation. "On my return home," he says, "on board the ship which brought us from Bordeaux, I met with a quiet and pleasant Anglo-Indian doctor, some time retired, old and matter-of-fact of manner, who was very full of the subject

---

[1] We deal in Chap. X. with the hypothesis that Lourdes is a centre of " Mass-Suggestion," and content ourselves here with some account of the cures which are effected at the shrine.

when once I opened it. Lourdes had been a
favourite study and a common haunt of his; and
he professed himself entirely unable to account
for many of the cases for which the evidence was
clearly too strong, in any known or reasonable
way. A French friend of his, he told me, suffered
from an affection of the eyes for which he had consulted the oculists. They had all agreed that it
was a well-known organic affection for which there
was no remedy, and that blindness must certainly
result from it. The Englishman from his own
experience could only confirm the sentence; but
moved by his friend's deep distress, he merely said
to him, 'Try Lourdes.' 'But I have no faith
in these things,' was the reply. 'No more have I,'
said the doctor. 'My faith is entirely suspended;
but there are qualities in the Lourdes cases which
I do not understand, not to be accounted for by
any explanation within our present knowledge.'
The Frenchman tried the waters. He went alone,
not as a member of any of the pilgrimages. And
after a few visits to the well the cloud passed
suddenly from his sight, and he was cured. The
affection did not recur. The Englishman examined
his eyes, and found all traces of the malady gone.
I tell the story as it was told to me, but the
character of my informant left me no room to
doubt its absolute truth. The strangest part of
the story was that, while thousands of the faithful
appeal in vain, this was no case of faith-healing,
but healing against the reverse of faith. 'All I
know is,' said the doctor, 'that in this especial case
anything like hysterical action was, and must have

been, conspicuously absent. But I can gather for myself no certain conclusion except the strengthening of my belief in agencies as yet quite unknown. There may be qualities in the water which cannot be analyzed.' 'But that,' I said, 'scarcely removes the wonder. It only shifts the ground. Why should the water which sprang from the earth after the reported " vision " act in this strange capricious way? It is the faith of others, not the patient's own, which is supposed to work these sudden cures from time to time, for purposes and meanings which are dark to us. Now, as of old, "the one is taken and the other left," as if, above and outside the ruthless and unresting forces of Nature, there were some Power at work which can, and does, set those forces aside for the hour and lend a world of meaning to the story of the Valley of Ajalon.' But it never did, and probably never will give any reason why, search and dive into the endless riddle as we may. These cures of Lourdes, for really to deny them is merely idle, may be no more miraculous in the stricter sense, if all were known, than the cable or the telephone. They may be merely the application of an unknown law. Then why the caprice of them? It looks, at all events, more like the setting of known laws aside, and it is there at present that the riddle of the healing lies. As to the mere question of the water, it is, I believe, true that the springs of Wildbad in the Black Forest, which bubble up about you as you lie upon a bed of firm white sand, have equally escaped the results of analysis."

This statement bears internal marks of genuineness, and in the absence of all guidance in formulating an explanation we may refer, with much diffidence and many reservations, to the widespread belief in guardian spirits as part of the more comprehensive belief in animism. On the supposition that the popular belief in the soul as man's invisible self has its correlate in reality, and that such soul on death persists in its individuality in some form or other—both strongly contested hypotheses—it would be not impossible that such a soul or souls, in the state which follows physical death, may be entrusted with the work of ministry for souls still in the flesh.[1] Further, it may be not impossible also that their knowledge is more profound and their power greater in matters which concern the causes of which our physical conditions are the effects—a third bare hypothesis. If it were allowable for the moment to suppose that these three hypotheses were not wholly irrational, we should at least be able to quote both pagan and Christian beliefs in their support. Moreover, most people would tell us that at times they seem to have been aware of contact with some unseen Being, to have heard words more or less unspeakable, and to have seen things for which ordinary knowledge has no explanation. Further, allowing as much as we like for "the long arm of coincidence," there would still, it seems, be left over signs of "a providence which shapes our ends," and orders the progress of the events which form at once our destiny and our character. Is it

---

[1] The reference here to the " soul," must be qualified by what is said in Chap. VII.

then, it will be urged, wholly irrational to accept, at all events provisionally, the hypothesis which finds expression in the saying that a good little angel sits up aloft to keep watch over the life of poor Jack?

It would be impossible to give all the apparently well-authenticated cases of "miraculous" healings that have taken place at Lourdes. Some of the more striking, however, will be enough to establish the claims made for Lourdes as a healing centre.

A Dr. Cochet of Avranches had in 1873 a patient, the Abbé Guilmin, aged sixty-seven, who had suffered since he was thirty from multiple abscesses on the left side of the breast, and had been for eight years under Dr. Cochet, as well as for eleven years under a Dr. Emile Fleury of Ducey. In 1876 the idea came to the Abbé to make a pilgrimage to Lourdes. The result is thus stated by Dr. Cochet—

"On March 6, 1876, he came to me and said that he was completely cured; in fact, the fistulous tracts which formerly furrowed the region of the malady were closed, and only a non-morbid swelling was left on the bones affected. The local lesion was perfectly cured, and besides M. l'Abbé Guilmin was in perfect health. Profoundly interested, I asked him for an account of this extraordinary cure, and he told me that after thirty years of suffering, exhausted by copious suppuration, at the end of his strength and almost sixty-seven years old, the inspiration came to him to make a neuvaine at the shrine of Our Lady of Lourdes, and at the end of it he felt himself relieved from his protracted sufferings, so much so that he was able on the same day to make a journey of forty kilometres. This relief was not accompanied by the exit of any fragment of diseased bone. ' I declare solemnly,' said Dr. Cochet, ' and on my conscience that this cure brought about under such conditions has no explanation in the facts of science, and in no way comes under the laws of pathology.' " Dr. Fleury bears the same testimony on the same date,[1] and adds that the cure had been progressive between 1873 and 1876, and was then complete.[2]

M. Georges Bertrin, Professor of the Paris Catholic Institute, gives a detailed account of the cure of a field labourer named Pierre de Rudder in 1875, whose leg had been broken six years before by a tree falling on it and crushing it. The result had been two open and suppurating sores which had become gangrenous; the tibia, or shin-bone, had in it a gap of an inch where it had been fractured, so that "the lower part of the leg could be turned in any direction. The heel could be lifted so as practically to fold the leg in half. The foot could be twisted until the heel was in front and the toes at the back." Rudder refused amputation, and Listerian antiseptics were hardly known. On April 25, 1875, three witnesses signed this declaration : "The undersigned declare that they saw on April 6, 1875, the fractured leg of

---

[1] March 6, 1876.

[2] Docteur Boissarie, *Lourdes, Histoire Médicale*, Paris, 1891, p. 200 f. ; Georges Bertrin, *Histoire Critique des Événements de Lourdes*, 1912, p. 553 ff.

de Rudder; the two parts of the broken bone pierced the flesh, and were separated by a suppurating wound an inch long. (Signed) Jules van Hooren, Edouard van Hooren, Marie Wittizacle."

The next morning (April 6) de Rudder set out from Jabbeke, his home, for Oostacker, a "cell" of Lourdes. There, sitting before the statue of the Blessed Virgin, his whole being became convulsed, he knelt down before the statue, discovered that he was actually kneeling, got up and walked round the grotto. His wife fainted on seeing him walking. On examination it was found that the bones were re-united, and the wound was healed. On April 15 thirteen of the principal citizens of Jabbeke, including two priests, the mayor, several aldermen and councillors, together with the Viscount du Bus, on whose estate the accident had happened, and who did not believe in miracles, and a M. P. Sorge, a free-thinker, signed the following declaration, which was sealed with the municipal seal—

"We, the undersigned parishioners of Jabbeke, declare that the shin-bone of Pierre Jacques Rudder, native and resident of this place, aged fifty-two years, had been so fractured by the fall of a tree on February 16, 1869, that every resource of surgery having been exhausted, the patient was given up and declared incurable by the doctors, and considered as such by all who knew him; that he invoked Our Lady of Lourdes, venerated at Oostacker, and that he returned cured and without crutches, so that he can do any kind of work as before his accident. We declare that this sudden and admirable cure took place on April 7, 1875."[1]

M. Henri Lasserre gives an account at great length of the cure of a Jeanne de Fontenay, who had been the victim of a carriage accident and under medical treatment for some years. For seven years she suffered violent pain in her viscera, and was for a long time unable to walk. Many remedies were tried, visits to Aix-les-Bains, hydropathy, and even a tentative visit in 1873 to Lourdes, where she obtained temporary relief. But her impotence coming on again, she went in the next year again to Lourdes, and there, on August 15, the Feast of the Assumption, she was instantaneously cured at High Mass, and walked and ran, taking her bed with her. The diagnosis of her case is given by Dr. A. Mangin of Baccarat, who testified on December 16, 1874, that her case had been medically diagnosed as "an organic lesion of the interior viscera," an affection which was evidently to be considered as "the beginning of all the nervous phenomena experienced by the patient, including the weakness of the lower members, which for a long time had rendered it impossible for her to walk, and had obliged her to keep her room, extended on a sofa or in bed." Dr. Lagoutte of Autun described the disease as a uterine affection, and affirmed that she "recovered her health completely and instantaneously, and that she could (January 31, 1875) use her limbs freely

[1] Georges Bertrin, *Lourdes, A History of its Apparitions and Cures*, 1908 ; *Histoire Critique des Événements de Lourdes*, 1912, pp. 239–267.

and without pain." Further, Mgr. Langénieux, Bishop of Tarbes, in whose diocese Lourdes is situated, has allowed a commemoration stone to be let into the stone floor of the Grotto of Lourdes, bearing this inscription—

15th August 1874
On the Feast of the Assumption
Of the Most Blessed Virgin Mary
Mlle. Jeanne-Marie de Fontenay
of the
Diocese of Autun
was cured.

And also in the Cathedral of Autun an ex-voto tablet was erected bearing an inscription which runs—

For ever,
The 15th of Every Month at Half-Past Eight in the
morning, A Mass of Thanksgiving
To Mary Immaculate,
In Gratitude for the Recovery
Of Mlle. Jeanne-Marie de Fontenay
Obtained at Lourdes
The 15th August 1874.

Though no special weight belongs to these inscriptions, and in spite of M. Lasserre's pious rhetoric and also in spite of the ambiguity of the medical diagnosis, no substantial reason exists for doubting that a cure was effected sufficiently remarkable to strike the spectators of it, and to impress the two doctors quoted. Dr. Mangin writes as a fervid Roman Catholic.[1]

An interesting figure in the literature of Lourdes

---

[1] Henri Lasserre, *The Miraculous Episodes of Lourdes*, tr. M. E. Martin, 1884. Dr. Mangin's testimony is given also by Georges Bertrin, *Histoire Critique*, p. 466.

is Adolphe Retté, who published the story of his conversion from free-thought to Catholicism in a book entitled *Du diable à Dieu*, which rapidly went through twenty-four editions. In 1909 appeared the ninth edition of his *Un séjour à Lourdes, journal d'un Pélerinage à Pied, Impressions d'un Brancardier*, in which he tells us how Lourdes drew him to walk from Belgium to the rock of Massabielle, and there to enrol himself among the brancardiers, or guild whose work of mercy it was to act as porters to carry the sick to the piscinæ. Among the cases he quotes is one of Louise Vergnac, a child educated in the orphanage at Bergerac, and attacked in her fourteenth year with a curious affection of the bones of her left foot of a tuberculous nature. This foot was amputated in 1901, but in 1904 the right foot began to show symptoms similar to those of the left, and amputation was again advised, but not performed, as the mother preferred to try Lourdes first. Retté then recounts, after the Abbé Foulard, professor at the petite seminaire at Bergerac (whose account he assures us is accompanied by convincing medical testimony), what took place. The "miracle" took place August 8, 1904, three years after her left foot had been amputated. After praying in the chapel of the hospital of Our Lady of the Seven Dolours and meditating on the Dolours, she is plunged into the bath. At first she feels as if her disease were excited to fresh activity, and for three or four minutes she suffers intense pain. Then suddenly a fresh feeling takes the place of what had seemed a boiling heat; she leaves the bath cured, and returns to the hospital. There the bandages are undone, and it is found that the swelling has gone, the skin is in wrinkles now that the limb is reduced in size. She eats well, and sleeps soundly all the night. Each year since her cure Louise goes to Lourdes to report herself to Dr. Boissarie and to return thanks for her cure. On one of these occasions Retté met her and ascertained from her that when she went to Lourdes she had no belief in the possibility of being cured. Her only regret is that she did not go sooner, and so save her left foot from the knives of the surgeons.[1]

Another patient who told Retté that she was cured contrary to her expectation was Noémi Nightingale, an English girl of fifteen years, who was cured of complete deafness May 21, 1908. Retté says he had read her dossier, but he prefers to relate her story as she herself gave it him in a letter. When she was four she had measles, which left her with growing deafness and a suppuration in both ears. In 1897 she was operated on by a Dr. Cumberbatch. The tympanum of her right ear was found to be pierced through an abscess, and she became more and more deaf, though hearing at first fairly well with the left ear. By 1907 she had become completely deaf, and understood by lip-reading only. She relates her cure quite simply. "Last Thursday, May 21, in the afternoon I was saying my chaplet at the Grotto for the souls in Purgatory. It was a quarter to seven when all at once I felt pain in my ears. Thinking it was not much, I said nothing. But the pain became

[1] *Un Séjour à Lourdes*, Paris, 1909, p. 205 ff.

more and more intense, so much so that I have never felt any like it in my life. It was real agony for four minutes; I thought I should faint; it seemed as if I were asleep and dreaming. I saw nobody, and I do not know what happened until they began to sing the Magnificat. That was the first thing I remember hearing. Naturally I asked what it was, not being able to believe that for a miracle I was cured. However, I was not mistaken; it was true, very true; I was cured." Dr. Boissarie assured M. Retté that the Bureau was satisfied that the cure was complete.[1]

But of all the marvellous cures reported at Lourdes none is more graphic or better attested than that of Gabriel Gargam. This man, who was in the French Post Office, was sorting the letters in an express train from Bordeaux to Paris on December 17, 1899, when another express ran into his train from behind, and smashed to pieces the carriage he was in. When he came to himself he was in the hospital, with wounds in the head and legs, and fractured collar-bone. These were, however, the least of his wounds; they soon were healed, but he was left paralysed from the waist downwards and suffering from disastrous internal disorders. Eight months afterwards he was unable to take any nourishment, and he was reduced to little more than a skeleton. His weight was 78 lb. The Orleans Railway Company meanwhile was being sued for damages, and the doctor who had been called in to report on the case gave his report on December 19, 1900. The

[1] *Un Séjour à Lourdes*, Paris, 1909, p. 213 ff.

ı

wounded man was declared to be suffering from "paralysis with contraction, anæsthesia of the legs and exaggeration of the tendon reflexes, especially in the beginning; epileptoid trembling of the foot; very pronounced muscular atrophy of the lower limbs, and redness with a tendency to bed-sores in the lower regions of the back. All the symptoms have appeared gradually; they constitute an affection of the spinal cord called amyotrophic lateral sclerosis. This diagnosis appeared to me to be the correct one, to the exclusion of other diseases, such as compression of the cord or hysterotraumatism." On February 20, 1901, the Civil Court decided that Gargam had been reduced by the Company to "the most pitiable of states," that he was "a perfect wreck of humanity with only his intelligence left unimpaired." It therefore awarded him an annuity of 6000 francs for life and an indemnity of 60,000 francs. This decision was upheld on appeal.

Gargam, however, grew steadily worse. He was an unbeliever, but merely to please his mother and family he consented to go to Lourdes, though expecting nothing. He refused to salute the crucifix when he came in sight of Lourdes. His mind remained free, cold and detached. He was put into the piscina. Nothing happened. He lost consciousness; came back to himself, stood up, walked a short distance, was taken to the Bureau, but not examined till the next day. *The Annales de N.D. de Lourdes* [1] says, "Gargam arrived on his stretcher wrapped in a long dressing-gown,

[1] xxxiv. 322.

followed by his mother, his nurse and several ladies from the hospital. He got up in our presence, looking like a ghost. His large staring eyes were the only living spots in his emaciated, discoloured face; he was bald like an old man, yet he was barely thirty-two years old." The next morning Gargam walked into the Bureau, and on examination it was found that the gangrene in the feet he had suffered from was gone, its scar alone remaining; he was extremely thin, and the muscles of the legs had gone. However he could walk, and he eventually recovered perfect health. In three weeks he put on 22 lb. in weight. "To-day he weighs 165 lb. He can bear the fatigue of long hours of hard work at the piscinas, though he feels a certain weakness in his back at the spot where Dr. Teissier supposed that a vertebra was pressing on the medulla." [1]

M. Henri Lasserre was himself the subject of a cure of an affection of the eyes—hyperæmia of the optic nerve—which prevented him, in 1862, from using them at all for writing or reading, and necessitated the use of blue spectacles with dark shields at the side. He recounts at length the circumstances which led him, on October 10 of that year, to order a little bottle of Lourdes water to be sent him to Paris, and to apply it to his eyes with a towel. "Judge," he says, "of my amazement, I might almost say my terror! I had hardly touched my eyes and forehead with the miraculous water

[1] Bertrin, *Lourdes, a History of its Apparitions and Cures*, pp. 263 ff. ; Retté, *Un Séjour*, p. 222 ff.; Jörgensen, *Lourdes*, 1914, p. 161 ff.

when I felt myself cured, suddenly, abruptly, without transition, and with such rapidity that in my imperfect language I can only compare it to a flash of lightning. . . . No, I could not believe my senses. So much so that I fell into the sin of Moses, and struck the rock twice. I continued to pray and bathe my eyes, not daring to put my cure to the proof. In about ten minutes, however, the vital energy that flooded my eyes left me no longer in doubt." A slight return of the malady shortly afterwards was put an end to by anointing with some oil from the lamp before the Sacred Face at Tours. "Towards the beginning of the afternoon," he writes, "as I was walking in the street on my way to business, I suddenly became aware that the feeling of heaviness had disappeared, and that the potent fluids of health had penetrated beneath my eyelids, revivifying the nerves and muscles in the region of the eyes." Twenty years afterwards, M. Lasserre asserted that since the day of his cure by Our Lady of Lourdes his sight had never ceased to be excellent.[1]

When we come to compare the nature of the diseases which are related as having been removed by Spiritual Healing in distinct and independent centres, we shall find them singularly alike. Meanwhile, it is interesting perhaps to note that the division Dr. Boissarie makes of those recorded at Lourdes is into (1) tumours and gangrenous sores, (2) organic maladies, and (3) functional troubles and nervous disorders. The case of

[1] Henri Lasserre, *The Miraculous Episodes of Lourdes*, 1884, pp. 282-356.

Rudder given above will serve to illustrate the first class, to which may be added that of François de Lavaur, who suffered from 1852 to 1871 from varicose veins and ulcers in the leg, and was cured in one night by the application of compresses steeped in Lourdes water. This cure was attested by three doctors named Ségur, Rossignol and Bernet as being "a most extraordinary fact and indeed supernatural."[1] A case of cancer related by Dr. Boissarie belongs to the same class—that of Raymond Caral, an excise officer, whose disease Boissarie had no hesitation in declaring to be malignant. He was cured in eight days by bathing his cancerous face in the water of Lourdes, and nothing was left but an almost imperceptible scar.[2]

To illustrate the second class we may take the case of P. Hermann, whose failing sight issued in glaucoma, for which the physicians saw no remedy but iridectomy. A visit to the Grotto at Lourdes, and a novena ending on All Saints' Day, cured him. "Since then," he says, "I write and read as much as I want to, without spectacles, without precautions, without effort, without fatigue. I fix my eyes on the light of the sun or on the gas without feeling the least injury; I have got what I wanted: I am completely cured." M. Boissarie himself testifies to the cure, and quotes the opinion of the oculist who diagnosed the disease.[3]

Bertrin gives an account of a girl born deaf and dumb. "At the age of twenty she put a few drops of Lourdes water into her ear on three

---

[1] Boissarie, *Lourdes, Histoire Médicale*, Paris, 1891, p. 157.
[2] *Ibid.*, p. 171 f.   [3] *Ibid.*, p. 149 ff.

successive days, and on October 11, 1872, she suddenly found she could hear and speak. Of course she had to learn her words, for language is not acquired intuitively. The family doctor, De la Mardelle, who examined her after the event, wrote as follows: "From earliest infancy, this young girl who was placed under my care offered every symptom of natal deaf-mutism. . . . On October 11, on her return from a pilgrimage to Lourdes, she instantaneously recovered the faculty of hearing. . . . The cure is certain and undeniable. The deaf and dumb girl can hear and speak."[1] The cases of Rudder and Gargam cited above will also serve to illustrate this class of cures of organic disorder. Moreover, Dr. Saint Germain testified—going beyond Dr. Boissarie—that a case of coxalgia cured at Lourdes radically and instantaneously "was not nervous coxalgia; it was a very real disease with grave articular lesion."[2]

There is the less need to dwell on the third class of cures, those of functional disorders, because the medical faculty admits to the full the actuality of cures by suggestion.[3] Bernheim says of it that "suggestion is a remedy which is almost exclusively functional. It may succeed in re-establishing disturbed functions, but cannot cure diseased organs." "Suggestion cannot re-set a dislocated joint, bring down a rheumatic swelling, or restore destroyed cerebral matter. The direct rôle of mind-healing

[1] *Lourdes, A History of its Apparitions and Cures*, 1908 p. 111.
[2] *Ibid.*, p. 122.
[3] See, *e.g.*, the discussion in the *British Medical Journal* of June 18, 1910.

with reference to organic lesion should not be exaggerated; it is limited. It cannot bring about resolution of inflammation, stop the growth of a tumour, or arrest the process of sclerosis. Suggestion does not kill microbes, it does not heal a gastric ulcer." And again : "Only what is curable can be cured. . . . Suggestion cannot restore what is destroyed." [1]

Further, it is an admitted fact that suggestion, like all natural forces, takes time to work out what it has to do, and that the length of time required varies directly with the gravity of the disorder. But unless the annals of Lourdes are untrustworthy, there the cures are, for the most part, or very often, instantaneous.

Again, it is urged by the advocates of Lourdes that suggestion is not used there, by which they seem to mean only that it is not used formally and specifically. For it is obvious that the whole circumstances form a vast mass-suggestion, in which the belief of other pilgrims comes in to fortify the nascent belief of the patient and his hearty hope of a cure.[2] Yet, on the other hand, as in the case of Gargam, this explanation of suggestion is manifestly inadequate, to say nothing of the fact that it goes beyond the possibilities of suggestion as laid down by so high an authority as Bernheim.

Attempts have been made to attribute the cures of Lourdes to certain natural properties in the water. But, apart from the facts that the greater

[1] Bernheim, *Hypnotism.*
[2] On this aspect of Suggestion, see Chap. X.

number of cures are wrought outside the piscinas, and that hydropathy is no monopoly of Lourdes, we have the report of M. Filhol, of the Toulouse Faculty of Science, who, soon after Lourdes became famous, analysed the water for the Municipal Council at Lourdes. His report was that "this analysis proves that the water from the Lourdes' Grotto is a drinkable water, very similar to most of the waters found in mountains whose soil is rich in limestone. This water contains no active substance capable of endowing it with marked medicinal properties; it may be drunk without inconvenience."[1] And in his letter to the Mayor of Lourdes, which accompanied this report, M. Filhol said : "The extraordinary effects which are declared to have been obtained by the use of this water cannot be, at least in the actual state of scientific knowledge, explained by the nature of the salts of which the analysis discovers the existence."[2]

The negative results thus obtained may be also extended without much risk of error to the oil taken from lamps, or to handkerchiefs, or other articles belonging to a saint and applied to the sick. Whatever the explanation may be, we seem at least precluded from seeking it in the hypothesis of some unknown force inherent in the water, oil, or other objects used as media of cure.[3]

[1] Georges Bertrin, *Histoire Critique des Événements de Lourdes*, 1912, p. 170.
[2] *Ibid.*, p. 171.
[3] " It is *not* true, a thousand times it is *not* true, that a bottle of water from a spring near which a girl saw a hallucinatory figure will by miraculous virtue heal a Turk in Constantinople ;

AN AMERICAN LOURDES

An American Lourdes is in great request at St. Anne de Beaupré, a village twenty-one miles from Quebec, where a chapel was built by the first French settlers in 1658 and dedicated to St. Anne, the mother of the Blessed Virgin, who showed her pleasure at the foundation of it by healing Louis Guimont, an inhabitant of Beaupré, of acute rheumatism in his loins. "Miracles" have been worked there since for two centuries and a half, and in token of them there may be seen on either side of the main doorway of the existing church (built in 1876, consecrated in 1889) "huge pyramids of crutches, walking-sticks, bandages and other appliances left behind" by those healed by St. Anne. Since 1892 the basilica has been in possession of a wrist-bone of St. Anne, four inches long, brought from Rome.

It also possesses the bone of a finger of St. Anne, first exposed in 1670, and in 1891 a bone of her hand was given by the Bishop of Carcasonne; in 1880 was given by Father Charmetant a fragment of rock taken from the grotto which was St. Anne's room during her mortal life. It has also the miraculous statue of St. Anne, round which the pilgrims kneel in prayer for healing; this costly statue replaces a more ancient statue in wood which is still preserved among the treasures of the church.

---

but it is true that on some influx from the unseen world—an influence dimly adumbrated in that Virgin figure and that sanctified spring—depend the life and energy of this world of every day." F. W. H. Myers, *Human Personality*, 1903, i. 215.

Like other healing centres, that of St. Anne de Beaupré has a holy spring which has been instrumental in "a crowd of marvellous cures. . . . Without doubt the water of these springs," says a pious Roman Catholic, "has not itself the power to effect these marvellous cures; but if God wills to make use of it as a means of working miracles, who would deny His power to do so?" As at Lourdes, the stream has been civilized and made to flow since 1876 into a large reservoir. In 1905 no fewer than 168,000 pilgrims visited the shrine, and the number seems to be steadily increasing. Unfortunately, it is difficult to get much information in England about this interesting shrine.[1]

The Case of Dorothy Kerin

Mr. Hilaire Belloc, in his fervid preface to Jörgensen's *Lourdes*, asks, "If what happens at Lourdes is the result of self-suggestion, why cannot men, though exceptionally, yet in similar great numbers, suggest themselves into health in Pimlico or the Isle of Man? It is no answer to say that here and there such marvels are to be

[1] I have not been able to get access to the *Annales de la bonne Sainte Anne de Beaupré*, which are published every month, nor to a work by l'Abbé Thomas Morel, priest in charge in 1661, who in 1668 published for the edification of the faithful an account of the miracles worked at Beaupré "of which he had been the eye-witness, or about which he was well informed." See Paul Victor Charland, O. P., *La bonne Sainte, ou l'histoire de la dévotion à Sainte Anne*, Quebec, 1904, and *Les trois Legendes de Madam Sainte Anne*, Quebec, 1898, by the same author; *Le Sanctuaire de la bonne Sainte Anne de Beaupré par un Père Redemptoriste*, 1904, and the note s. v. in the *Catholic Dictionary*, vol. i. p. 539.

found. The point is, that men go to Lourdes in every frame of mind, and are in an astonishing number cured." The answer to Mr. Belloc's question is threefold. In the first place, it is not contended (here, at all events) that auto-suggestion, or even suggestion in general, is competent to account for the "miracles" of Lourdes. In the second place, Mr. Belloc offers us a false alternative when he bids us choose between self-suggestion and "the best influence there is for men (I mean that of Our Blessed Lady)," for, to say the least, a third power and perhaps a fourth may be assigned with even greater plausibility, as we shall suggest presently. In the third place, it is a gross exaggeration to say that men are "in an astonishing number cured" at Lourdes. Father R. J. Clarke does not claim more than two per cent. of miraculous cures, and in a Roman Catholic account of the return of the English pilgrims from Lourdes this year we are told: "'There was expectancy among the crowd. The crowd wanted to hear of the marvellous happenings in the little Pyrenean town of Lourdes. There were questioning whispers and much excitement, and probably a little disappointment; for the news, when the excitement was gone and the facts were considered, was this: there had been no cures; there had been many cases in which relief was experienced by the sufferers, but no cures to which medical knowledge would give countenance."[1]

But we may go further and say that Lourdes

[1] *The Universe*, June 12, 1914. The same absence of cures marked the previous year.

has no monopoly of curative power, and that what takes place there has taken place in Jersey [1] and Herne Hill—for Mr. Belloc is clearly using "Isle of Man and Pimlico" in a Pickwickian sense. The "Herne Hill Miracle" seems as well authenticated as any miracle performed at Lourdes. Dorothy Kerin was a young woman of twenty-two, who, for about seven years, had been seriously ill, and through most of that time bedridden. On May 22, 1906, she was admitted to the Box-Grove Sanatorium at Reading, and the diagnosis on admission was: "Hysteria, hysterical vomiting, hæmatemesis, vicarious in origin." In January 1907 she was discharged "in excellent health." In January 1908 she spent three weeks in the same sanatorium by invitation, and was then active and cheerful, with lungs perfectly healthy.[2] In 1908 we have a report from her then medical attendant which is also given on the same page just quoted —he had her under his observation for about six months. She complained of pain after food and vomiting, but had healthy heart and lungs, had no cough and no evening rise of temperature. Analysis revealed no sugar, blood or albumen in the urine, and the doctor was clear that then she suffered from neither consumption nor diabetes.

On June 26, 1908, Dorothy Kerin was admitted to the St. Bartholomew's Hospital, and there treated for gastritis. She was discharged on August 30, and declared to be "strong and well." But on returning home she had a relapse and took to her bed. One medical man who examined her

[1] See Appendix D.
[2] British Medical Journal, March 9, 1912, p. 545.

at this period "satisfied himself that the invalid had no symptom or physical sign of pulmonary tuberculosis," and also "he dismissed the idea that hysteria or malingering accounted for the condition." Another medical practitioner who attended her during the same period thought that no tuberculosis could be found, and he fell back on hysteria as the disease. In January 1909 she was examined in the out-patient department of Mount Vernon Hospital, without any definite result. The next month she went to St. Peter's Home of the Kilburn Sisters, where she developed alarming symptoms, and was taken home by her mother to die, as the mother supposed. Even then her medical man thought that hysteria was the cause of her trouble.

After this, however, things grew worse, and her medical attendant from February 1910 to February 1912 diagnosed her disease decisively as pulmonary tuberculosis with severe hæmorrhage, aggravated by what seemed to be peritonitis. She suffered from great fall of blood-pressure, extreme exhaustion, inability to retain food, with general collapse. She was officially notified under the Compulsory Notification of Consumption Act.

On the evening of February 18, 1912, at about 9.20 p.m., her relations were gathered round her bedside to see her die, when suddenly she was heard to say, "I am listening." She then sat up in bed, rubbed her eyes, opened them, and smilingly said that she had had a wonderful vision, in which she had been told by a Voice that her sufferings were ended. She then insisted on having her dressing-gown brought, got out of bed, walked round the room, and after examination showed that she had no symptoms of tuberculosis at all. This is her own account of her vision—

"I always wished and prayed that I might be resigned and happy in doing what God might will, but I never once asked Him to make me well. . . . Sometimes I used to wonder why God permitted it, but I was always certain that I should know some day . . . but I did not think I should ever realize it in this world, but I do now, don't I? I never endeavoured to help myself by suggestion of any kind. I used to try and take all the food and medicine I could to try and get well, and to use all the means that God had sent, but if they failed I did not bother. When I used to partake of the Holy Communion, it was not with any thought that it might possibly be the means of making me well some day. . . . I always spent a good deal of time in intercession. . . . I always used to feel an inexpressible nearness to God, especially at night when I could not sleep, and I never felt alone. I never had any particular dreams, and never dreamt that I was well." About Christmas 1911 she had a vision in a dream of a lady in white who picked her a lily, but this led to nothing. When she found she was restored to health on her third vision she was filled with "an unspeakable thankfulness" impossible to be described. "I knew it was not merely a dream that had restored me to health. Of course it was not a dream. I thought God had brought me back to do some great work for Him, and I thought He had performed this wonderful miracle to teach people in that way, because they could not be taught and shown in any other way. . . . When I woke up on Monday morning I felt as if I had never been ill before. The beautiful light and vision was on my mind all the time I was asleep. It all seemed quite natural that I should get up. . . . I think it shows that God closes the mortal eyes sometimes, so that the eyes of the soul should be opened, because if my mortal eyes had been open perhaps I should not have seen and heard [the visions] so clearly." [1]

It is easy, of course, for a critic to doubt whether the last medical man who diagnosed this case was not mistaken, but in view of the symptoms described the doubt seems unreasonable. In any case Dorothy Kerin was seriously ill, and was thought by all, including herself, to be at death's door. Or it may be objected that hers was a case of the mimicry of phthisis by hysteria. But, in the first place, the mimicry would seem to have caused what it began by mimicking. And, in the second place, even hysteria is a serious and well-marked disease, and the words of the *British Medical Journal* in another connection are worth noting. "We are in full agreement with Sir Clifford Allbutt when he says that a careful study of all reported cures of a miraculous kind proves that they all—palsies, convulsions, and the rest—are, and have been, cures of one disease and of one only—namely, hysteria. Surely we may here say, with Sir Thomas More: ' Marry, this is somewhat ! ' The cure of hysteria is the cure of a very real disease." [2]

[1] Edwin L. Ash, *Faith and Suggestion,* 1912, where the case is discussed.

[2] *B. M. J.*, March 9, 1912, p. 554.

When, however, we speak of hysteria as a very real disease, all that we can mean at present is that it is a disease of uncertain origin with very serious disorders of manifestation. "We do not know anything about its nature, nor about any lesions producing it; we know it only through its manifestations, and are therefore only able to characterize it by its symptoms, for the more hysteria is subjective, the more it is necessary to make it objective in order to recognize it." [1] But a disease, whatever its ætiology, is a very serious malady which produces as symptoms such evils as paralysis, spasms and contractions of muscles, loss of voice, perpetual cough, rapid breathing, vomiting, hiccough, retention of urine, painful joints, fits, catalepsy, hystero-epilepsy, anæsthesia, hyperæsthesia, astasia and abasia, to say nothing of the havoc it works in the realm of the will and emotions. If, then, the vision of a beautiful angel radiating light, saying, "Dorothy, your sufferings are over, get up and walk," was sufficient to cure this very real disease of hysteria alone, no good ground exists for belittling it, or for placing it in any different category from that which embraces the "miracles" of Lourdes. The only difference there is, is that in the one case the glorious personage who works at Lourdes said who she was at one of her early appearances, while in the other case she did not, but the difference is not to the discredit of the later vision.

[1] J. M. Charcot and Pierre Marie, in Tuke, *Dict. of Psychol. Med.*, vol. i. p. 628.

CHAPTER VI

CHRISTIAN SCIENCE

OF all the movements of modern times which come under the general heading of Spiritual Healing, that known as Christian Science is the most striking both for the more than Papal autocracy which governs it and for its material extension. It is difficult to know which is the more marvellous, the grotesqueness of its accepted doctrines, the credulity of many of its followers, or the failure for so long of orthodox religion and medicine to see the essential truth latent in its activities.

Mary A. Morse Baker was born in New Hampshire, July 16, 1821, of farmer stock, and of a father who was "a tiger for temper and always in a row." [1] Masterful, interfering, quarrelsome, prejudiced and narrow-minded, the father reappeared in the child. In her early days disciples of Mesmer and Andrew Jackson Davis and the Shakers familiarized her with the idea of healing outside the regular channels. [2] When she was twenty-two she married a George Washington Glover, who died six months later, and three months after his death a son was born to him. Nine years later she married Daniel Patterson, [3] an itinerant dentist, and as Mrs. Patter-

[1] *Life of Mary Baker G. Eddy and History of Christian Science*, by Georgine Milmine, 1909, p. 7.
[2] *Ibid.*, p. 23 f.   [3] *Ibid.*, p. 33.

son she was afterwards remembered as a woman of
"ungovernable temper and hysterical ways," [1] and
her life till 1866 was spent in "ill-health and dis-
content." In 1862 she first made the acquaintance
of a healer named Phineas Parkhurst Quimby,
a clock-maker by trade, a cultured and upright
man, and she became one of his patients and
disciples. His *Science of Health*, with its doctrine
of the divine man incorporated in another man, the
first being Truth, Goodness and Wisdom, and the
second being Ignorance, was the germ out of which
Mrs. Eddy afterwards developed her system.
Quimby died January 16, 1866, and soon afterwards
Mrs. Eddy had revealed to her directly from God
her "Science of Metaphysical Healing."

After P. P. Quimby's death Mrs. Glover (as she
called herself then) spent about nine years in
moving from place to place and in brooding over
Quimby's ideas. Her first book was published in
1875, but in 1870 she had persuaded a youth of
twenty-one, Richard Kennedy, to go into partnership with her, he doing the practical healing and
she supplying the theory. Kennedy testified of
her that she held even then of her pupils that "so
long as they believed in a personal God and the
response to prayer, they could not progress in the
scientific religion." On January 1, 1877, she
married one of her pupils, Asa Gilbert Eddy,—he
died in 1882, of what his wife described as
"arsenical poisoning mentally administered," and
was actually valvular disease of the heart.

In the first edition of *Science and Health*, Mrs.

[1] *Plymouth Record*, July 16, 1904.

Glover took Quimby's gospel of healthy-mindedness, threw in a few ingredients from the Shakers' tenets, flavoured the whole with Andrew Jackson Davis, and, adding touches of her own, claimed for the whole direct inspiration and revelation. The immunity from criticism thus secured has been loyally maintained by her trusting followers, with some striking exceptions, down to the present time. This book of 1875 has been thus decribed : [1] "Even after her eight years' struggle with her copy, the book as printed in 1875 is hardly more than a tangle of words and theories, faulty in grammar and construction, and singularly vague and contradictory in its statements. Although the book is divided into chapters, each having a title of its own, there is no corresponding classification of the subject, and it is only by piecing together the declarations found in the various chapters that one may make out something of the theories which Mrs. Glover had been trying for so long to express." In this book, however, is contained the peculiar philosophy which goes by the name of Christian Science and forms the basis of the "treatment" given by Christian Scientists.

So far as an orderly philosophy can be constructed out of *Science and Health* it is one which may be called an idealistic monism. Mind is All and All is Mind. All that exists is an immortal Principle which is defined as Spirit, God, Intelligence, Mind, Soul, Truth, Life, but "there is no life, truth, intelligence nor substance in matter— matter is moral error—is the unreal and temporal."

[1] *Life of Mary Baker G. Eddy*, p. 178.

For the next seven years Mrs. Eddy was engaged in attempts to build up in Lynn a nucleus of believers in her doctrine, and was involved in numerous law-suits which were generally regarded as discreditable to her and to her newly discovered religion. Moreover, she seems to have become obsessed by the delusion that "Malicious Mesmerism" was being continually practised against her by a band of enemies of whom Kennedy was the chief. In October 1881 eight of her nearest friends and principal supporters sent her the following letter, which is quoted here as a succinct statement of the difficulties thrown in the way of *Christian Science* by Mrs. Eddy's own character and actions—

"We, the undersigned, while we acknowledge and appreciate the understanding of Truth imparted to us by our Teacher, Mrs. Mary B. G. Eddy, led by divine Intelligence to perceive with sorrow that departure from the straight and narrow road (which alone leads to growth of Christlike virtues), made manifest by frequent ebullitions of temper, love of money, and the appearance of hypocrisy, *cannot* longer submit to such Leadership; therefore, without aught of hatred, revenge or petty spite in our hearts, from a sense of duty alone to her, the Cause and ourselves, do most respectfully withdraw from the Christian Science Association and Church of Christ (Scientist)." [1]

This and similar resignations left Mrs. Eddy with no more than a dozen students in Lynn, and

[1] *Life of Mary Baker G. Eddy and History of Christian Science,* by Georgine Milmine, New York, 1909, p. 276.

soon after she retreated to Boston, having to all appearances failed in her mission, and this at the age of sixty-one.

Soon after their arrival in Boston, Mr. Eddy died of organic disease of the heart, or of what Mrs. Eddy declared was "malicious mesmerism," which she chose to identify with arsenical poisoning applied mentally. A Mr. Calvin A. Frye,[1] however, was found who could act as Mrs. Eddy's factotum in the work which now at last began to grow under her hand. The "Massachusetts Metaphysical College of Boston" gained an increasing number of students; these were sent out to practise, and each acted as a new centre of missionary enterprise. The *Journal of Christian Science*[2] was founded in 1883, and in 1886 there appeared a new edition of *Science and Health* revised by the Rev. J. H. Wiggin, a cultured Unitarian minister. And as the number of students increased so did their belief. *Science and Health* slowly crept up to an equality with the Bible, and Mrs. Eddy with Jesus Christ, she proclaiming the Motherhood of God and he the Fatherhood, while what she called "M.A.M.," that is, Malicious Animal Magnetism, was the equivalent in Boston of Demonology in Palestine. On the other hand, criticism started up without and within her band of inherents, and in 1888, out of two hundred members of her Church in Boston thirty-six sent in their resignations. But though Boston might be the centre of her movement, its strength was now too widely established to be endangered by disloyalty even in the centre.

[1] *Cf.* Milmine, p. 293.　　　[2] *Ibid.*, p. 312.

Churches were now established in many towns, and societies not yet organized as Churches in many more. Moreover, Mrs. Eddy contrived to make herself autocrat of the Church which in 1894 began to arise in Boston, as the mother-church of the Christian Science movement.

From that time to her death, Mrs. Eddy lived in retirement at Pleasant View in Pleasant Street, which she had bought, and from there she exercised a general superintendence over an organization which was now deep rooted. She was at length, by force of character and astute generalship, the undisputed autocrat of the vast society she had brought into being.

It seemed necessary to give this brief sketch of the career of the founder of Christian Science if we are to do justice to the principles and methods of that science. We may pass by as irrelevant the criticisms passed on her personal character as being the true child of her father and in addition a neuropath. Both may be true without affecting the value of her teaching. Similarly, her indebtedness to Quimby is valuable only for purposes of analysis, and does not affect the value of her method any more than the authorship of Shakespeare's plays affects their character as literature. The question at issue is not whether Mrs. Eddy was all the saint her admirers say she was or the victim of morbid egoism as her enemies allege. It is not whether her "Revelation" was purely from above or whether Quimby, Evans, Davis and others supplied the materials for Mrs. Eddy to put together. The question is whether *Science and*

Health is true, whether its main principles are in accordance with the nature of Reality. And a second question may be raised. Given the truth taught by *Science and Health,* do the cures ascribed to the practice of it flow directly from it, or are they cures which might as well follow from some similar but different method, such as prayer on the part of an orthodox believer? And, further, is Christian Science justified in obliterating the distinction made by orthodox medicine between "organic" and "functional" disorder?

It is not to the purpose to dwell on the confusion of thought, or want of literary skill of so much of *Science and Health* as Mrs. Eddy was responsible for. Mark Twain has said all that need be said on this head and it does not help the main issue very much. What this is may be best made clear by quoting Mrs. Eddy's own words in *Science and Health with Key to the Scriptures* (I use the edition published by A. V. Stewart in Boston, 1912). The following state axiomatically her faith—

"Christian Science reveals incontrovertibly that Mind is All-in-all, that the only realities are the divine Mind and idea." But as she goes on to say that "this great fact is not, however, seen to be supported by sensible evidence until its divine Principle is demonstrated by healing the sick and thus proved absolute and Divine," it seems clear that Mrs. Eddy herself does not regard her revelation as intuitively perceived but as rationally induced. We are referred to cases of healing given as evidence in her "Fruitage," at the end of the volume. Yet she says : "I won my way to absolute conclusions through divine revelation, reason and demonstration."

Again : "The three great verities of Spirit, omnipotence, omnipresence, omniscience,—Spirit possessing all power, filling all space, constituting all Science—contradict for ever the belief that matter can be actual. These primeval verities reveal primeval existence as the radiant reality of God's creation, in which all that He has made is pronounced by His wisdom good." Hence she "beheld as never before the awful unreality called evil."

Further, Mind as immortal is distinguished from "mortal mind," the latter being defined as "sick and sinful humanity," and matter is defined as "the subjective state of what is termed by the author mortal mind."

And finally, we are given, as the translation of ordinary terms into "scientific," *God* as meaning : Divine Principle, Life, Truth, Love, Soul, Spirit, Mind; *Man* as meaning God's spiritual idea, individual, perfect, eternal; *Idea* as meaning an image in Mind, the immediate object of understanding. On the other hand, we are given as "the scientific translation of Mortal Mind " that it is in the first degree depravity, being physical only. Then *physical* is defined as : Evil beliefs, passions and appetites, fear, depraved will, self-justification, pride, envy, deceit, hatred, revenge, sin, sickness, disease, death. In the second degree we find evil beliefs disappearing and we get the Moral. The *Moral* is defined as : Humanity, honesty, affection, compassion, hope, faith, meekness, temperance.

In the third degree we rise to Understanding which is the *Spiritual,* and this is defined as : Wisdom, purity, spiritual understanding, spiritual power, love, health, holiness. So "mortal mind disappears and man as God's image appears." And to illustrate the principle thus set forth we are assured that Jesus "showed that diseases were cast out neither by corporeality, by *materia medica,* nor by hygiene, but by the divine Spirit casting out the errors of mortal mind."

In the above extracts the substance of Mrs. Eddy's philosophy is contained, and the rest of her book and all her other writings either vary or elaborate the theme. And the first obvious remark on the statement of this philosophy is that it is a crude setting of a great truth which was only half understood by the author. Long before her day Bishop Berkeley had set out in his idealistic philosophy the non-reality of matter, and a greater than he, Plato, had done the same two thousand years earlier. And according to one of the latest champions of Christian Science, Mrs. Eddy did not mean by her philosophy anything more than orthodox idealism in general means. "Christian Science has never taught," he says, "that matter is not real to the human consciousness, but that it is unreal in the sense of ultimate reality, and in the sense that it forms no part of God's spiritual creation, which is the only real or actual creation." [1] But if this is the defence put in it can only be said that it is a double-edged weapon. If Mrs. Eddy

[1] *A Plea for the thorough and unbiassed Investigation of Christian Science,* by an Enquirer, 1913, Dent, p. 23.

meant no more than this the Christian Science movement would have died in its birth. But it was the something more which gave it its vitality, and this something more was the belief both of Mrs. Eddy and her followers that sin, disease and death were the products of "mortal mind"—that is, of the false thinking done by men, and that they could be actually and experientially destroyed by such true thinking as is expressed in the affirmations "I am God, I am infinite Truth, I am Love, I am Goodness." It was no question of "ultimate reality" which agitated Boston, but of getting rid there and then of an actual and troublesome delusion. And the delusion is said to be destroyed by an affirmation about Spirit being the sole form of Reality. But what if this be but another delusion? By what canon are we to distinguish truth from falsehood? The schools may be quarrelling still on this question, but Mrs. Eddy is satisfied that her system is known by its fruits. It works, and therefore is true. Even then the question still remains whether the cures effected are so effected that to Christian Science alone can the credit be given. We will endeavour, before we have done, to point out that Christian Science can justly point to Spiritual Healing as the results of its working, but that there is no reason for saying that no other method can be effectual.

It is argued in support of the sole existence of Spirit that God is perfection, and that therefore, "He is not and cannot be conscious of evil, or of the material world as we know it, for in order to be so He would need to possess the imperfect human consciousness to present to Him wrongly His own perfect spiritual creation."[1] But what this writer does not see is that "perfection" is quite compatible with finiteness, and that therefore a creature ringed about with "matter" may be as perfect in its degree as God is *ex hypothesi* infinitely perfect. The ephemeral insect subject to speedy death, and living only to propagate its kind, may be perfect in its place. Man subject to "mortal mind," the prey of delusions and narrow vision and poor aims, may also be perfect in his present stage of evolution.

An instance of this use of the term perfection may be taken at random in the following sentence which occurs in a note to the Article on Evolution in the *Encyc. Brit.*, XIth edn.

"Kant, for example, held it probable that other planets besides our earth are inhabited, and that their inhabitants form a scale of beings, their *perfection increasing* with the distance of the planet which they inhabit from the sun."

"Christian Science teaches," however, we are told, "that God being perfection, all His creations must be perfect because they are expressions of Himself. Therefore He did not and could not create a sinful man, or a man that could become sinful."[2] Then we are to suppose that since there are all around us, as an inexpugnable fact, men who have become sinful, they are either not men in the transcendental sense of Christian Science, or that as phenomenal beings they owe their existence

[1] *A Plea for the thorough and unbiassed Investigation of Christian Science*, by an Enquirer, p. 28.
[2] *Ibid.*, p. 33.

to some power which is not God. Mrs. Eddy appears to hold both, for she does not regard man as he is as true man, and she ascribes to "mortal mind," that is to fallen man's mind, the creative power of calling into being pain, disease and death. But this last is but the mediæval doctrine about the Devil, and Mrs. Eddy herself is a terrible example of the power of "mortal mind" over herself, for during the greater part of her adult life she was obsessed by a devil of her own creation, her dreaded M.A.M.—malicious animal magnetism. But apart from this, even supposing that "sinful man" is no creature of God's thought, where did "perfect man" get the idea from to which he proceeded to give phenomenal existence? Did he not derive it ultimately from his own being but call it up as a new creation? In this case we have the Devil over again but now in a human form. Or did he derive the material for his creature from the treasures lying within or without him? In this case God Himself is ultimately responsible for the evil man has brought about. In either case Christian Science philosophy is hopelessly discredited as a philosophy. Yet we are told that "the whole case for Christian Science rests upon the assumption of the truth of its philosophy and religion. Every cure brought about by Christian Science is the direct result of mental work in accordance with its teaching. Prove that its philosophy is unsound and you destroy the whole fabric."[1] This enshrines a familiar fallacy. The philosophy may be

[1] *A Plea for the thorough and unbiassed Investigation of Christian Science*, by an Enquirer, p. 10.

unsound and yet the cures may follow from another and an unsuspected cause.

A second criticism which may and must be passed on the philosophy of Christian Science is that it shows no awareness of what is perhaps the most important outstanding problem of all philosophy, that of Time. It is the problem of how the One which dwells in Eternity becomes the Many whose activities are determined by sequence. It is quite true that philosophy in general has no solution of this riddle any more than Christian Science, on its own showing, has of the origin of Evil. But modern philosophers are all agreed that in some sense Evolution, that is, a process in Time, leads on organic life from perfection to perfection, from a lower grade of perfection proper at one stage to a higher grade proper at another stage. And a common illustration of this is the doctrine of epigenesis or the addition of the higher perfection by the "successive differentiation of a relatively homogeneous rudiment into the parts and structures which are characteristic of the adult." But the only evolution Mrs. Eddy seems ever to have thought of was that of the gradual triumph of her philosophy over all the existing delusions born of mortal mind. Had she, however, been reminded that all things even now are perfect in their degree, and rise to higher and higher perfection indefinitely under the gentle pressure of the Life-impulse and under the form of the Time-order, she would have been given a doctrine which would have made unnecessary most of what she wrote about the genesis of Evil and God's necessary ignorance of it.

A third fatal flaw in her system was due to her inability to distinguish between a system of know-ledge and a system of reality. She assumed that they were the same. If man, she taught, would cast off the shackles of delusion and prejudice he would rise from the part to the whole, would see and know as God, or infinite Intelligence, and his thought about things would be the thought of God ; he would stand at the centre of the universe (as Hegel essayed to do), and be as God, knowing good and evil, not in experience but in their roots, and so would be master of their effects. Mrs. Eddy did not see that what she called illusions were the attempts of "mortal mind " to read the riddle of the Universe from the place where it found itself, and that its readings were not delusions (which is what she meant by illusions) but illusions in the strict sense, that is, partial fragments of truth promising in due time to bring forth larger portions and there-fore more of Reality. Imperfect knowledge does not mean that the knowledge is not about the Real, and is not valid so far as it goes ; it does mean that all knowledge in every stage is methodological, an aid to our understanding and to our practice, but not constitutive of the Real. Mrs. Eddy, on the contrary, confusing ontology (a word she uses) with methodology — reality with knowledge— assumed that Spirit could be perfectly known by men in her generation, and that perfect knowledge carried with it perfect power. And the first of these propositions rests on a confusion and the second on a one-sided anthropomorphism.

In the fourth place, Mrs. Eddy was quite unaware

that Spirit, Life, Intelligence, Love are all terms expressing a mental construct of "mortal mind" as truly as Matter is another such mental construct. Our primary consciousness is not from two minds, one immortal and one mortal, but only one mind. And whether the concept which this one mind forms be valid or not cannot be determined by constructing *a priori* two categories, one for immortal Mind and another for mortal mind, and then bundling our experiences into one or the other at the bidding of hedonism, as Mrs. Eddy does, but by patiently piecing together the scattered fragments of our human experience in order to fill in as best we can an outline of the ideal in that ultimate synthetic thought which lies and perhaps will for ever lie beyond our reach, calling us on and on as the *Ewig-weibliche*, always making us happy, and yet never fully contenting our longings for the living God.

But so far we have contented ourselves with following the lead of Mrs. Eddy's own apologists, which stakes the whole of Christian Science praxis on the validity of its philosophy. In doing this, however, these apologists seem to be doing her a disservice. For it not unfrequently happens that people stumble on a truth which is greater than their apprehension of it, and no confutation, therefore, of the discoverer's explanation is necessarily effective against the Truth itself. What is more, Mrs. Eddy won all her success by using the one weapon which she denounced in her philosophy as evil, first, last, midst and without end. It is not too much to say that the whole Christian Science organization is the product of Mrs. Eddy's own "mortal mind." The fiery energy with which she pursued Kennedy, Spofford, Arens and everybody who ventured to thwart her; her dogged determination to be successful at all costs and to rule over the society she had formed; her numerous lawsuits; her obsession by the fear of animal magnetism, and the final result of all her struggles for unquestioned authority over the whole movement, all go to illustrate the fact that, whatever might be the worth of her theories, her practice at all events, affords a signal instance of the extraordinary power of "suggestion" when adequately applied. The uniqueness of immortal Mind may be the content of the Christian Science gospel, but it was mortal mind which gave it driving power and moulded and knit together a world-wide society. Græcia capta cepit victorem. Mortal mind after all came by its own, and its trophy is the Church of Christ (Scientist).

But to say this is not to account for the one important fact about Christian Science. Mahomet won, it is said, his adherents at the sword's point, but where did he get his sword from? Mrs. Eddy exercised to the full the powers of her mortal mind through suggestions given strongly and sometimes volcanically throughout her life. But what is the value of the doctrine she suggested? What exactly is the Truth by which Christian Science effects its cures? The answer is to be found unquestionably suggested in the philosophy, even though it is not precisely the philosophy itself.

This Truth is, in the first place, effective, though in a much more limited area than Mrs. Eddy knew.

On the face of her philosophy the processes of Nature, physical death and every form of disease were under the control of the Christian Scientist who surrendered his mortal mind and became 'mortal Mind instead. As Lyman P. Powell puts [1] "Mrs. Eddy, for the encouragement of the faint-irted who find matter a stubborn fact, indis-suuble even in the crucible of Christian Science, pleads guilty at one time or another to having raised the dead, ' brought out one apple-blossom on an apple-tree in January when the ground was covered with snow. And in Lynn demonstrated in the floral line some such small things.' " And the late much respected Dr. Edward Everett Hale wrote : "Mrs. Eddy said to me that I might cut through the main artery of her arm and that she would stop the effusion of blood by an exertion of will." [2] In the chapter headed "Fruitage" in *Science and Health*, she tells of a patient being cured who had lost one lung (p. 624); of another who had "what the doctor called consumption in its last stages" (p. 623); valvular heart disease (p. 608); a broken bone (p. 606); kidney disease (p. 662); and an incurable disease of ten years' standing (p. 682). And indeed Mrs. Eddy boldly claims for Christian Science that it is as applicable to organic as to functional disorder. Her words in *Science and Health* (p. 176) are—

"Should all cases of organic disease be treated by a regular practitioner, and the Christian Scientist

[1] *Christian Science : the Faith and its Founder*, p. 111. New York, 1907.
[2] *Op. cit.*, p. 246.
L

try truth only in cases of hysteria, hypochondria and hallucination? One disease is no more real than another. All disease is the result of education, and disease can carry its ill-effects no farther than mortal mind maps out the way. The human mind, not matter, is supposed to feel, suffer, enjoy. Hence decided types of acute disease are quite as ready to yield to Truth as the less distinct type and chronic form of disease. Truth handles the most malignant contagion with perfect assurance."

From the above passages it is clear that Mrs. Eddy claimed for Christian Science at least healing power over all forms of disease, whether "organic" or "functional." It would be perhaps as arrogant and rash to say that Spirit cannot, or will not some day, cure organic disease, as it is to say that at our present stage of evolution we can safely eschew orthodox medicine for Christian Science in "cases of pyloric obstruction, gastric ulcer, dilatation, congenital malformation or cancer of the stomach," to say nothing of carious or broken bones, of destroyed nerves or amputated members.

But the field of "functional disease," it may be said, still remains, and it may be an even larger field than is ordinarily supposed, and perhaps the field where most of the suffering due to illness is to be found. But, on the other hand, it is extremely doubtful whether the distinction between "organic" and "functional" disease is anything better than a rule of thumb, or at best a convenient way of discriminating slight disorders from grave disorders. As Rudolf Arndt says: "If we keep in mind that there is no function without an organ, and that every function is but the product of the action of the latter, and must vary according to the nature of the organ, we cannot possibly doubt that there are organic changes in cases in which the functions are altered, however slightly. From a large experience we shall derive the conviction that there can be no difference between the so-called functional and organic diseases, but that when the former develop and when disorders of function have existed for a longer or shorter time, they can have sprung only from organic changes." [1] So Fagge, while admitting that there is a not inconsiderable number of disorders which force themselves into notice by the pain or discomfort they occasion and yet disclose after death no alteration of organ or tissue even under the microscope; and after saying that outside toxic disorders there still remain defects of secretion, of movement and of innervation which we must regard as purely functional, yet goes on to say that "although we may still distinguish between *organic* or *structural* diseases attended with recognizable morbid changes, and *functional* diseases in which no such lesion is found, yet the progress of science is continually transferring maladies from the latter to the former class. So that the distinction between functional and organic disorders is, though convenient, not fundamental." [2]

Further, the trend of medical science is to go

[1] Tuke's *Dictionary of Psychological Medicine*, vol. ii. art. " Neurasthenia," 1892.
[2] C. H. Fagge, *Text Book of Medicine*, 4th ed. 1901, vol. i. p. 3.

behind the symptoms to the disease, to seek for the anatomical lesion which occasions the disease and for the pathological process which has caused the anatomical lesion. The steady pursuit of the ultimate disturbing force marks the progress of medicine, and in the main, until recently, medical science has been content to believe that ultimately the ætiology of disease is to be located in the matter of the living body, even where in special cases its instruments refuse to disclose it. But the use of hypnotism made during the last thirty years, and the increasing importance assigned to mind in fostering both health and disease, tend to weaken this appeal to matter as the final arbiter.

This tendency, however, does not necessarily carry us beyond the realm of mechanism, for, as was suggested above, mind may be regarded as (when in operation) a higher and more delicate kind of machine. We are not, therefore, led necessarily any nearer to Mrs. Eddy's declaration that "when divine Science overcomes faith in a carnal mind, and faith in God destroys all faith in sin and in material methods of healing, then sin, disease and death will disappear." Nor are we any more disposed by this change in medical outlook to accept Mrs. Eddy's assertion that she had cured what is termed organic disease as readily as she had cured purely functional disease, and with no power but the divine Mind.

The gulf is still fixed between the belief in Mechanism, physical or mental, which distinguishes medical science and the belief in Life which characterizes religion. And so far as we can see the two must be still regarded as at all events methodologically distinct, for we have no knowledge or skill to construct a bridge which will make the two one.

It is here where Mrs. Eddy's distinguishing merit is to be found. She made religion an instrument of healing, or rather she found Quimby and many before him healing by suggestion, by touch, mesmerism and hypnotism, by mental healing in general, and she lifted their doctrine and methods into a religion. And her religion rests on the assertion that Life, as opposed to Mechanism, can heal all diseases, to which she adds that it can do so here and now if we know how to get hold of it. It is the office of Christian Science to tell us how to get hold of Life here and now. To these two claims we shall probably be safe in saying that the first is true and the second false. Life, which is God, can no doubt secure or restore health and banish all disease. But, if we may use a scholastic distinction, it is one thing to say *simpliciter* that Life can do this, it is another thing to say so *cum suppositione.* God, we must suppose, has committed Himself to the cosmic process, and is bound, therefore, by what that process has brought about, as He would not have been bound without that process. This implies that while God, or Life, could, speaking *simpliciter,* bar out every approach of disease, or drown it in the flood of His creative Life, yet on the *supposition* that tissues and organs have behind them a long history written in their submission to an infinite network of cause and effect, He cannot now drive out disease at will unless He

is prepared to abrogate arbitrarily the Law of
Causality. In other words, Christian Science
stakes its theoretical existence on the miraculous—
that is, the arbitrary, or supplanter of the existing
order, and this modern science in general is agreed
in regarding as a superstition.

To illustrate this point let us remember the Law
of Compensation, a law which rests securely on a
sufficient induction. This tells us that the development of an organism in one direction is invariably
purchased by loss in another. Man, for example,
has developed along the line of Mind or Reason,
and he has had to pay the price for his attainments
in the loss of certain bodily functions, notably in
the sense of smell and in sensibility to movements
in Nature which the plant world and lower animals
retain. The crustaceans, on the other hand, to take
one example, have not developed as man has done
and so they retain a power man has lost. If one
of their claws is broken off, they can grow a new
one. Man cannot, or at all events does not. But
in the assertion that Christian Science can achieve
even this feat there is implicit the almost incredible
belief that it can reverse the whole evolutionary
process of thousands of years in a moment, and this
without paying the necessary price in the abandon-
ment of our mental achievements. But is there any
valid reason for supposing that we can, through
invoking the Life, secure the power of having our
cake and eating it at the same time, of retaining
our Reason and regaining our early animal capacities—that is, of gaining what would be to us a
new power without paying the price demanded by

the Law of Compensation? Of course, a single instance of a new leg being grown under the instigation of Christian Science in place of one amputated would cause us to revise at once our question. But, so far as is known, Christian Science alleges no such case, and yet it should be in a position to do this unless its claims are made more modest.

The truth, in fact, is that its claims are well founded, though they are valid in a narrower field than its most fervent adherents would have us suppose. For practical purposes we may accept the distinction between functional and organic disease, and say that in the former class Christian Science not only can do but has done much beneficent work, worked many cures, and brought self-control, renewed hope and a braced and invigorated physical system to numbers of afflicted persons. And it has done this by mental suggestion as the immediate means, and by evoking as the remote means the health-giving forces of the divine Life which inheres in all mechanism, physical or mental. Moreover, it has somehow come to operate on so large a scale that it has impressed the imagination of the civilized world and made it impossible for it ever again to forget the paramount right of Life in the omnipresent coalition of Life and Form. To Christian Science, therefore, we are all debtors, and any criticism we pass on our creditor has its sole justification in the duty we owe to truth to ascertain precisely the amount of our debt. And in the end we find that the debt is a real debt and a large debt, though not so large as Mrs. Eddy was

disposed to think. It is enough to point to the fact
that the wave of desire for Spiritual Healing which
has over-run two continents derives the greater
part of its volume from the contribution made by
Mrs. Eddy and her followers.[1]

[1] The fundamental tenet of Mrs. Eddy's philosophy is to be
found in P. P. Quimby's *Science and Health,* with its distinction
of the divine man incorporated in a lower man. This truth,
however badly stated, is the key to Spiritual Healing, and those
who are repelled by the grotesqueness of Mrs. Eddy's phrase-
ology may be recommended to study Carl du Prel's statement
of it in his *Philosophy of Mysticism,* or the two volumes of
Mr. F. W. H. Myers's *Human Personality.* It is the same
truth which alone can correct the pessimistic conclusion of
Schopenhauer's philosophy ; and it forms the presupposition
without which the teaching of Jesus Christ remains incoherent.

CHAPTER VII

SPIRITUAL HEALING AND THE BODY

IF Spiritual Healing is to be properly given a place among the activities of our world, an attempt must be made to show that there is nothing in its nature which makes its existence antecedently improbable. And this means that we must show that human nature is such that it *can* give rise to Spiritual Healing, and then, when we have shown that it *can*, there will remain only the task of selecting a sufficiency of evidence to show that it *does*, and afterwards the further task of finding out *what* it is.

The analysis of human nature most widespread is that which, following St. Paul, makes man to be threefold, consisting of body, soul and spirit. But there are serious doubts for assigning any place to the intermediate thing called the Soul. It is not a thing, indeed, which modern psychology knows much about, for it prefers to deal with Mind instead. But even so, Mind takes on a twofold aspect according as it is turned inwards towards pure thought or outwards towards sensation. So that the difficulty we meet when we ask about the nature of the Soul is not done away with by substituting Mind for it. Soul may be considered abstractly as being on one

side Will, on another Thought.[1] And each of
these, again, may be higher or lower as we direct
Will or Thought to what is more spiritual or more
material. It would seem better, therefore, to say
that what we are is a union of spirit and body, and
that Soul is but a convenient name we give to
denote succinctly our present mixed condition, in
which the union of spirit and body is still imperfectly realized.

It will be best to begin our inquiry by taking the
body first. This is often spoken of as being a
physical body because it is compounded of elements
drawn from the world of physics. Or sometimes
it is described in terms of mechanism, because it
does work, just like any machine, which can be
measured in foot-pounds and represented in the
curves of the statistician or the zigzags of the
hospital sick-bed. But, in truth, both these forms
of description are merely abstract, and may be,
therefore, misleading. For they leave out of
account that which differentiates the body from
physics and chemistry, and from all machinery that
we are acquainted with. They forget that the body
is an animated body, is while it lasts the possessor
of life, is, in short, an organism. Not that there
is any stigma cast on the body by describing it

[1] Benedetto Croce, as is well known, discards Feeling as a
third with Thought and Will, except as a name for the states of
pleasure and pain. "Feeling," he says, "has been the indeterminate in the history of philosophy, or rather the not-yet-
fully determined : the *half-determined*." (*Philosophy of the
Practical*, 1913, p. 25.) He appears to allow, however, a place
for Feeling as the undifferentiated Power which, when it enters
the world of Space and Time, becomes differentiated into
Thought and Will.

as a machine, if we keep in mind what sort of a machine we mean. "The adult mind is coming more and more to be treated as, at least *inter alia*, a shopful of machines."[1] For our present purpose what Spinoza says (*Ethics*, III. Prop. ii. proof) is of importance. After asserting that the mind and the body are one and the same thing, which, now under the attribute of thought, now under the attribute of extension, is conceived, he goes on to say : "No one has thus far determined what the body can do, or no one has yet been taught by experience what the body can do merely by the laws of nature, in so far as nature is considered merely as corporeal or extended, and what it cannot do, save when determined by the mind. For no one has yet had a sufficiently accurate knowledge of the construction of the human body as to be able to explain all its functions. . . . Again, no one knows in what manner, or by what means, the mind moves the body, nor how many degrees of motion it can give to the body, nor with what speed it can move it. Whence it follows that when men say that this or that action arises from the mind, which has power over the body, they know not what they say, or confess with specious words that they are ignorant of the cause of the said action and have no wonderment at it." Spinoza then points to the phenomena of sleep-walking, as showing that bodily powers may be enhanced by the cessation of waking consciousness, and to the fact that "when the body is inert the mind likewise is inept for

[1] B. Bosanquet, *The Principle of Individuality and Value*, p. 177.

thinking." And his general conclusion is that "the decision of the mind and the desire and determination of the body are simultaneous in nature, or rather one and the same thing, which, when considered under the attribute of thought and explained through the same, we call *decretum*, and when considered under the attribute of extension and deduced from the laws of motion and rest we call *determinatio*." It is not within the free power of the mind to remember or forget anything, and we are not free in our volitions any more than "the infant which thinks that it freely desires milk, the angry child which thinks that it freely desires vengeance, or the timid child which thinks that it freely chooses flight."

To state the capacities of the mind in terms of machinery will seem to many to go back from teleology and to degrade mind to the level of matter. But in point of fact such a process is not so much the degradation of mind as the exaltation of body. Is not an "actual soul" which is highly trained and definitely habituated a better soul than one which is governed by impulse alone? or is every step in the cultivation of intelligence a backward step? Few would answer this last question in the affirmative.

The fact is that the dualism which assigns teleology to the mind (or soul) and mechanism to the body is unwarranted. Mechanism is not fossilized teleology, but is, instead, that through and in which teleology works. For the mind of everybody is a complex system of "dispositions," just as the nervous system is. We do not think or will in entire independence of our mental and volitional habits, but in complete interdependence of the one on the other. If the mind, then, is thus of the nature of a mechanism, the body is also teleological in its very structure. For the purpose which we so generally assign to mind would not be in mind at all but for its partnership with an external matter. "Teleology," it has been well said, "does not come out of the empty mind; it is the focusing of external things together until they reveal their internal life."[1] It may be going too far to say that "all definite differentiation of the soul belongs to the body, and that all tendencies and capacities are transmitted through bodily arrangements," though it might be contended that the soul first creates many of its differentiations and is afterwards bound by them, and that its tendencies and capacities are less transmitted than limited by its body's arrangements. On the other hand, it is certainly false to say that the body is the soul's passive partner, doing just what it is told or compelled to do by a power not itself. It is not so much a physical body, but what St. Paul called it, viz. a psychical body, that is, a body which is alive with a life which is its own, and is not a lodger who is free to depart when he will, or a soldier quartered on his host by the arbitrary fiat of a stranger. The relation of the soul to the body is not so much that of a sailor to a boat, or a charioteer to his chariot, as that of the music to the strings of the harp while it is being produced, behind both harp and its music being the harpist.

[1] B. Bosanquet, *The Principle of Individuality and Value,* p. 166.

In this sense, then, we say that the man is an organism in which efficiency and degree of value depend on the perfection of the mechanism as much as on the energy of the Life-force which drives the machinery. For the more highly developed any mechanism is, the more capable it is of being adapted to new needs as they arise. The more easily so heterogeneous a complex can be thrown out of work, the finer is the work it can do when it is in working order. Also the care it demands is in proportion to its delicacy and the balance of its parts. Thus a wheelbarrow, as the simplest of tools which use wheels for communicative motion, will go on for months without being oiled, while a ship's engines require constant care. This analogy may serve to illustrate one aspect of Spiritual Healing.

For all illness is caused in the last analysis by a breakdown somewhere in the machinery of the human organism, be the cause of that breakdown what it may. That machinery has a marvellous power of self-readjustment, and will make heroic efforts to keep itself running by adapting itself to the abnormal demands made on it. When, however, the Mind sets itself to learn the nature of the trouble, its cause and the method of its cure, and then proceeds to do what is necessary for restoring health, we may, without doing violence to words, call this a case of Spiritual Healing, even though it be exercised in a quite rudimentary fashion.

But the truth just insisted on, viz. that of the possession by the body of powers it does not as a rule get credit for, is useful to our inquiry in another respect. It will help to clear away something of the mist which clings round the term "subconscious." It might be thought, to hear some people talk, that the sub-conscious side of our nature was not only greater in the volume and importance of its activities, but also higher in dignity and in its place in evolution than our reflective waking or every-day consciousness. For it has control of all our involuntary movements, such as the breathing of the lungs, the beating of the heart, the ingestion of our food and the excretion of waste products through the sympathetic nervous system. And, what is more, it acts in dreams and under anæsthetics; it is the organ of inspiration, creation or invention; and when ordinary consciousness is stilled its activities are continued.

Under the name of subliminal Self the late Mr. F. W. H. Myers included "all that takes place beneath the ordinary threshold, or say, if preferred, outside the ordinary margin of consciousness," [1] all that for some reason never emerges into that "supraliminal current of consciousness which we habitually identify with ourselves." [2] This subliminal consciousness is not discontinuous or intermittent. It possesses faculties, *e. g.* telepathy, clairvoyance, clairaudience or telæsthesia, which are unknown to the supraliminal consciousness. It can so control the organism as, *e. g.* to produce blisters in response to suggestion, or the stigmata of a St. Francis, and this "control over the organism is more potent and profound than supraliminal, and

---

[1] F. W. H. Myers, *Human Personality*, 1907, p. 14.
[2] *Ibid.*, p. 15.

is exercised neither blindly nor wisely, but with intelligent caprice." [1] The phenomena of somnambulism, moreover, show that not only is the *influence* of the subliminal self over the organism greater than that of the supraliminal, but its *knowledge* of the organism is also more profound. In the case of "Hélène Smith," discussed by Prof. Flournoy in his *Nouvelles Observations sur un cas de Somnambulisme*, there appeared every kind of automatic irruption of subliminal into supraliminal life. "Phenomena of hypermnesia, divinations, mysterious findings of lost objects, happy inspirations, exact presentiments, just intuitions, teleological automatisms" [2]—all these marked the séances at which Hélène was the medium. And if anybody cares to pursue further his inquiry into the wonders of the sub-conscious self, he will find ample material offered him in such a work as Carl du Prel's *Philosophy of Mysticism*.

Here it seems necessary to discriminate and to hesitate some doubts. We may exclude here the one sense of "sub-conscious" which has a scientific value and precision, that used by professed psychologists. Its founder was Leibniz, who explicitly charged the Cartesians of his day with holding for nothing the perceptions which were not apperceived, just as the vulgar hold for nothing bodies not reported on by the senses. Herbart then distinguished between presentations which did not pass "over the threshold"—to use his phrase, now become well known—and those which did. When

---

[1] F. W. H. Myers, *Human Personality*, p. 151.
[2] *Ibid.*, p. 281.

we are talking in public, for example, our being engrossed in our subject does not prevent the attitude of our hearers from impressing itself on our minds. But it is only afterwards that these weak impressions are brought into the field of consciousness to be focussed there. So long as they do not get this favoured treatment by attention they remain "sub-conscious" for want of intensity. But between the strong focussed presentation in attentive consciousness and the weak "sub-conscious" presentation in the margin there is a continuity which forbids us to place the latter anywhere save in the same category as the former. It belongs to the conscious region in spite of its Cinderella inferiority.

The hypothesis, moreover, of a sub-conscious self seems on other grounds unable to carry all the load it is called on to bear. A power whose activity ranges from the control of the beating of the heart to the finding for Saul of his father's asses may be used as a mask for quite disconnected things. How does it leap from its physical activities over the whole range of ordinary consciousness into the world of knowledge of facts which lie wholly beyond this waking consciousness? Thus it would seem likely that quite disparate things have been lumped together, and that, if we are to follow the lead of writers like Mr. Myers, we ought to speak of sub-conscious, conscious and super-conscious. "Consciousness, discernment, is another means which spirit uses in order to secure its own essential progress. Spirit itself is supra-conscious, and matter, it may be said, is infra-conscious. Consciousness is a feature of the middle stage, and is

M

conceived of as vanishing when it has served its purpose in providing a free passage for spiritual activity." [1] This description of M. Henri Bergson's philosophy would substitute for sub-conscious the unconscious, and insist that within matter potential consciousness is present, but is held back and rendered impotent by the inertia of matter itself.

The sole useful denotation, then, of the term sub-conscious is that which limits it to the habits of mind or body which the subject has inherited from its past. Samuel Butler has insisted with insight and force on present faculty being the memory of all we have done or suffered in the ages that have elapsed since we were a mass of undifferentiated protoplasm. A habit, says St. Thomas, after Aristotle, is "a certain disposition according to which the thing disposed is well or ill disposed either in itself or towards something else." [2] That is to say, experience impresses on each individual subject a readiness to respond more readily to some external stimuli than to others. Thus Prof. De Morgan, who read algebra as others read a novel, started in life with a mathematical habit. The young Pope who lisped in numbers because the numbers came, the Wunderkind who plays sonatas at three, or speaks a foreign language at five years of age, must be supposed to have a past which has produced a "habit of the mind" and made these marvels possible. So far, then, from our starting with a mind like Locke's *tabula rasa*,

---

[1] J. M'Kellar Stewart, *Critical Exposition of Bergson's Philosophy*, 1911, p. 53.
[2] *Summa Theologica*, i. ii., qu. xlix., art. i.

a sheet of white paper, we find it more like a slab of infinitely variegated and streaked marble, in which the coloured veins *are* the marble itself.

It may, of course, be objected here that the need of postulating such a complex of latent powers is rendered impertinent by the principle of imitation, in accordance with which we begin as children to learn, and continue as adults also our education. But this omits the necessary factor of the capacity for imitation, which makes it possible for us to teach a dog to jump through a hoop and impossible ordinarily to make a chair walk. We are not specially concerned here to contend that the "habitus" is to be traced back to pre-existence of the soul, or to the hypothesis of germ-plasm. It is enough to point to the fact that we do possess a complex of powers and capacities, whether of mind or body, and that it is to this complex we refer when we use the term "sub-conscious."

But in this case we are apt, as experience shows, to forget one important thing about this complex, and that is that it is illegitimate to restrict it to the phenomena of mind, as contra-distinguished from those of body. In this connection the two are indistinguishable, for both are integral parts of one organism, that is, of one mechanicalized whole, through which Life plays in accordance with the laws of the machine. When, for example, reference is made to the phenomena of somnambulism, as when Mr. Myers, for example, asserts that "the somnambulic personality is discerned throughout as a wiser self," [1] we can only reply that in the

[1] *Human Personality*, 1907, p. 157.

first place there is no evidence that the somnambulistic subject enjoyed any "representation" at all apart from its appropriate organ, and in the second place that the hypothesis is quite intelligible which says that all the conditions (though not all the causes) of somnambulism can be found in the living body itself. That living body is a machine which for two-thirds of its existence is run under the control of consciousness, but at other times goes on running at a lower speed uncontrolled, or only partially controlled, by consciousness.

Let us emphasize once more—for this is necessary to the proper understanding of one form of Spiritual Healing—the fact that the mind also is on one side of the nature of a machine, as well as the body. Nor is this to be regarded as any slight on mind, but is merely the statement of a fact. The mind is not at liberty to think arbitrarily or capriciously, as if under no necessary conditions. On the contrary, it is bound by the essential laws of Logic, whether these be correctly understood or not. Thinking in contradiction of those laws is not so much bad thinking; it is not thinking at all. But this is only to say that the mind is but a mechanism after all, even though it be a higher mechanism than some others. Moreover, not only is it seen to be formally mechanical; it is also a mechanism materially. For much of its content, perhaps we should say all its content, is of the nature of a highly elaborated network of past experiences woven so as to be able to incorporate at all times all events or actions which fresh experience brings. But, again, these new experiences are never "pure."

Simultaneously with their presentation there are also presented automatically cognate experiences from the inner treasure-house of "memory." The two sets at once blend, and so the wonderful mechanism of mind is from moment to moment modified and enriched. But it remains a mechanism all the time.

But while insisting that Mind and Body are each a mechanism we state only half the truth. Life is the other half, and in mentioning "Life" as the chief force with which the medical practitioner has to deal we are in presence of the most fascinating of all problems, viz. the mystery by which simpler forms become complex, and the most baffling because Life is the principle of indeterminateness. We do not know what Life is; all we can say is that it is a Force which, when in a relatively permanent association with matter, sets up certain processes which issue in appropriate phenomena. But we are not in a position to set limits to those processes by assuming that we have exhausted their possibilities. In fact, there is good ground for supposing that radio-activity is characteristic of Life, and that, therefore, what we know is but a fragment of the total activity of Life. We can say, for example, that Life does not within our experience change stones suddenly into bread. We are not justified in saying that it cannot. We may affirm that we do not know how to walk on water when in its liquid state, but we can hardly affirm that there is any inherent contradiction in the act. There was a time when a man would have been revered as a god had he flown through the air as aviators now do, and certainly David Home would have run great risk of being burned for witchcraft in the Middle Age if he had been seen to indulge in levitation and float through the window and back again without any visible means of subsistence.[1]

The acceptance of telepathy by men like Sir Oliver Lodge [2] opens up to Science a new field of inquiry. And it would seem that for the present no better term than "Telepathy" can be devised to collocate the carefully observed facts of the transference of thought from mind to mind apart from the ordinary means of communication. We will take one or two examples to illustrate the nature of the Life which seems to operate in dream-consciousness. In a lecture given at the London Polyclinic by Dr. T. Claye Shaw, he said : "To my own knowledge the following occurred : A man went down to a river to fish, and was not seen again; the river was diligently searched for many days, but no trace of him was found. Then a keeper's daughter had a night vision—a dream, if you like—that she saw the body in a certain pool which she named; and there, as a fact, the body was found.

"Of course, the girl knew the river, had heard

---

[1] See the evidence of the Master of Lindsay in the Minutes of the Committee of the Dialectical Society published in 1893, p. 214.

[2] "It appears that we can operate (on each other's minds) at a distance, without apparent aid from physical organ or medium ; if by mechanism at all, then by mechanism at present unknown to us." (*Man and the Universe*, p. 45.) Mr. Myers supposes telepathy to be a fundamental law of the spiritual world corresponding to gravity in the physical. (*Human Personality*, 1907, p. 31.)

of all that had been done in the way of searching, knew of the reward for the finding of the body, and doubtless had thought much upon a subject which caused intense local excitement; but may not that very excitement have rendered her susceptible to actual movements which must have occurred and which, as it were, accidentally perhaps came within the sphere of her cognition? No, you will say, it was a mere coincidence, or a judgment founded on reasoning that this particular pool had perhaps not been searched. Well, it may be so, but, on the other hand, there was no certainty that the man was in the river at all. During his act of going to the pool and of falling in there must have been a great disturbance of medial agencies, which only awaited the necessary receptor for their recognition.

"A man with good eyesight might have seen the occurrence a quarter of a mile off; a hawk with better eyesight might have seen it twice or three times the distance. Why may not this girl have been sensitive to medial vibrations which could only affect a receptive agency of a definite reciprocity?" [1]

Those who are interested in the question as to the nature of those dreams which seem to involve "psychical invasion" will find abundant material

[1] *British Medical Journal*, June 18, 1910, p. 1473 f. Again : "It may be within the reader's knowledge that I regard the fact of genuine thought-transference between persons in immediate proximity (not necessarily in contact) as having been established by direct and simple experiment; and except by reason of paucity of instance, I consider it as firmly grounded as any of the less familiar facts of nature such as one deals with in a laboratory." Sir Oliver Lodge, *Proc. Scy. Psych. Res.*, ii. 189.

in *Phantasms of the Living*,[1] and in the selection
from them which appears in Mr. Myers's *Human
Personality*.[2] But as space prevents the use of this
material we must content ourselves with evidence
of dreams in modern times which were directly
concerned with the healing of disease. Nobody
will benefit more from a study of the phenomena
of dreams than the medical man himself, unless,
indeed, it be his patient, for, according to Aristotle
(verified by Freud), "the expert among physicians
say that great attention is to be paid to dreams,"
because to definite diseases correspond definite
dreams.[3] So Maudsley says [4] that "dreams sometimes have a truly prophetic character in regard to
certain bodily affections, the early indications of
which have not been sufficiently marked to awaken
any attention during the mental activity of the day,
or to do more than produce an obscure and form-
less feeling of discomfort, but which nevertheless
declare themselves in the mental action of dreaming,
when other impressions are shut out. When the
disease ultimately declares itself distinctly in our
waking consciousness, then the prophetic dream,
the forewarning, is recalled to mind with wonder."
Thus we are told [5] of Aristides, whose coming
tumour was announced by a dream of a bull wound-
ing him in the knee; of Conrad Gessner, whose
dream that he was stung by a serpent was the
precursor of a plague-boil on the breast; of a man

---

[1] Ed. by F. W. H. Myers and E. Gurney, 1886.
[2] 1903, vol. i., Appendix to chap. iv. pp. 369-436.
[3] *On Prophecy in Sleep*, chaps. i. and ii.
[4] *Physiology and Pathology of the Mind*, 1867, p. 241.
[5] Carl du Prel, *Philosophy of Mysticism*, i. 197.

who refused to have an ulcer in his leg opened by
the knife, and suddenly woke from a dream in
which the ulcer had been cut to find that it had
burst of its own accord. It is also suggested by
Du Prel that the delusions of insanity are due to
bodily disorders which cause a mental condition
not wholly unlike the phenomena of dream-life.
Some bodily abnormality excites the sensory nerves,
these arouse dream-images, which in their turn
react on the bodily affection, and the whole process
may issue in motor activity of the muscles, such
as twitching of the limbs or of the face, or, in
extreme cases, in somnambulism.

There is nothing "supernatural" in dreams of
this character. All that they show is that in the
dream condition, whether of ordinary deep sleep
or in sleep hypnotically produced, a different kind
of consciousness obtains. In this second consciousness the inner sensibility is exalted, and the condition of the bodily organs is seen more clearly
and more profoundly than by the waking consciousness. Hence this inner sensibility is able to
diagnose the condition of its bodily organs, and
(since it is not devoid of will and intelligence) to
prescribe the method of cure. Du Prel can hardly
be accused of groundless speculation when he
correlates the *vis medicatrix Naturæ* with the *vis
medicatrix animæ*, seeing that it is the same unconscious (to us) Power which works in both. Anybody who considers the marvel of the process in
spring-time, when the trees put on their green
robes once more, may also understand the cognate
marvel of the restoration of health to the body by

the operation of the same unconscious Life-impulse. Nature, within and without and all about us, is ever in its own way at work building, repairing, breaking down and rebuilding, and of this unceasing process in us we get reports, all too scanty, but precise enough, from the phenomena of dreams and hypnotism.

But still the question remains as to the *modus operandi* of this hidden force, and to this question two answers are given. The first is that of the liberation of the soul from its bodily envelope, a theory which finds much asseveration in Theosophy, but insufficient evidence. According to this theory, the soul in deep sleep is able in its "astral" to quit the body and visit distant places, have intercourse with other matter-free souls, and see and generally experience things which while imprisoned in the body it is shut off from. In this condition, it is important for our present purpose to note, it has the power of conveying light and life to others in ways which ordinarily are blocked, but in deep sleep are opened.

A variant of this theory is that favoured by Spiritualism, which attributes the phenomena of the dream-life to the invasion of the secondary consciousness by souls from the other side. The only difference in substance between these two theories is that the one sees the efficient cause of dreams in souls temporarily liberated from the body which belongs to them, while the other sees it in souls which have shed their physical envelope and passed over to the world of shades. Both hold the theory of σῶμα σῆμα, that the body is a tomb in which the soul is imprisoned, and both, therefore, look to freedom from the body as the pre-condition of a higher and more powerful life.

The second answer to our question lies nearer to our hand, and comes from those who feel instinctively that the body is as truly an instrument as a hindrance. They point to the fact that in deep sleep the central nervous system sends in no reports from the external world, and that waking consciousness for the time is at rest. Since, however, a secondary consciousness is active, which is aware of what goes on within the organism, and to some extent of much that goes on outside the organism, they are led to inquire whether there exists any other nerve-system which can serve as the organ of this secondary consciousness in the same way that the central nervous system serves the primary consciousness of open day. They suggest as the organ required the sympathetic nerve-system. This position, however, seems more precarious than its supporters allow for, seeing that the progress of anatomical science has shown that the sympathetic system is less independent of the rest of the nervous system than it was formerly thought to be. The central nervous system with the peripheral nervous system alone do the work of transmuting afferent nerve-impulses into efferent nerve-impulses. This reflex action lies outside the sympathetic system.

On the other hand, the sympathetic system conveys efferent impulses to the muscles and also to the glands, while the cerebro-spinal system conveys them to the striated or voluntary muscles only. And the name *autonomic* is sometimes used to embrace all those efferent nerve-impulses which are not directly due to the central nervous system. Roughly speaking, then, the sympathetic system is the system of the involuntary in our organism. Its post-ganglionic fibres communicate with the whole of the alimentary canal from the mouth to the rectum, including the glands and blood-vessels; with the generative organs, the skin and the iris muscle and blood-vessels of the eyeballs.

We ought perhaps to go a step further and attribute our acquired habits to the sympathetic system as their organ. We walk and talk, certainly, without calling into play that intense form of consciousness we call attention. We may assume, then, by analogy that the voluntary muscles are not stimulated, but that the nerve-work is taken on by the involuntary muscles under the direction of the corresponding nerves. "Our nervous system grows to the modes in which it has been exercised" [1]; what appears in the lower animals as instinct appears in man as acquired habits, and in both cases a suitable nervous mechanism is developed as the organ of the instinct or the habit. And if we remember that the sympathetic nervous system is biologically an earlier formation than that of the cerebro-spinal, we shall be forced to regard it as the depository of all those quasi-reflex actions which the brain hands over to it to carry out when once the way to do them has become familiar.

This brings us round by another way to the

---

[1] W. B. Carpenter, *Mental Physiology*, 1874, p. 339 ; James, *Principles of Psychology*, 1890, vol. i. p. 110 ff.

conclusion arrived at earlier in this chapter, viz. that the sub-conscious is a term which should be restricted to the mechanism of habitual processes in living bodies, and should not be stretched so far as to cover the phenomena of deep sleep, of dreams or of hypnotism. When we are conscious our impulse is concentrated on the central portion of the field of consciousness, but we are also sub-consciously aware of much which lies further and further from the centre, and we hand over the work of utilizing this large sub-conscious material to the already fully developed sympathetic nerve-system. How well it does its work is well known when it suddenly reports the solution of a mathematical problem, or the nature of a disease, or the character of a person. It has noticed small details which escaped the "awareness" of consciousness, and has through its complex machinery worked them over and finally produced a rational result.

But in saying this we have, it will be observed, reached a conclusion which implies the action of something more than automatic nerve-movements. We have been forced to postulate the decisive action of some form of intelligence, differing in its mode of action from that which is called conscious. In other words, the nervous system, which, though fundamentally a unity, is yet differentiated into two for practical purposes, finds as its correlate a Mind which also is fundamentally one and yet acts in two markedly different ways. And, on the whole, it would seem that the conscious mind depends for its normal working on the cerebro-spinal nervous system, and that what we must call the super-conscious works through both this and the sympathetic system. For sanative, restorative and reproductive purposes its organ is the latter, and it is through this latter that the higher class of dreams is constituted. The importance of this fact to Spiritual Healing is too plain to need further elaboration. Its difficulties, however, disappear when we recollect that the real agent in either case is not the ego, whether conscious or unconscious, but the transcendental Subject which belongs to the world of Reality and uses in the world of Appearance the mechanism of mind and body—which mechanism has the character, not of dualism, but of identity.[1]

If, then, we have no option but to regard our phenomenal mind and body as two aspects of an organism all of whose activities are mechanically controlled, and therefore mechanically intelligible, we are constrained to add, in view of our inexpugnable sense of Freedom and of the facts of dream-consciousness, that we are not exhausted by the deliverances of our conscious Self. Behind the speech which fires is the orator; behind the poem the poet; and behind the human machine is the divinely-free Self. If we may borrow an illustration, we may say that the Self is the centre of two

---

[1] "When we say that an organism exists in a certain environment, we mean that its energy, or some part thereof, forms an element in a certain system of cosmic forces, which represent some special modification of the ultimate energy. The life of the organism consists in its power of interchanging energy with its environment—of appropriating by its own action some fragment of that pre-existent and limitless Power." F. W. H. Myers, *Human Personality*, 1903, i. 215.

concentric circles, the smaller of which represents our waking consciousness, the larger that whole world of our secondary consciousness, whose limits still remain to us unknown. The seat of this secondary consciousness is our transcendental Self, whose native home is in the intelligible or eternal order, whose working instrument in daily life is the empirical self as determined by the animated body in which it finds itself; in a sense, indeed, *is* the soul-body we use. It is not, however, the real Self, but only its counterpart, or its counterfeit presentment, its ἀντίμιμον πνεῦμα. The real Self is Mrs. Eddy's "immortal mind," St. Paul's "Christ in us," the "Thinker" of the Hindu, the "est Deus in nobis" of Ovid,[1] the "soul filled with deity" of Plotinus.[2] This "transcendental Subject" is the organizing principle of our two-sided empirical self, and when it is allowed to exercise its heavenly powers in an unusual degree we get inspiration, inventive power, superhuman fortitude or saintliness. When it is physical or mental recuperation that is required the agent in bringing it about is this "Higher Self," and we call his work, when we see it, Spiritual Healing.

[1] Est Deus in nobis, et sunt commercia cœli :
Sedibus ætheriis spiritus ille venit.
Ovid, *De arte amandi*, iii. 549.
[2] *Enneads*, vi. 9. 9.

CHAPTER VIII

SPIRITUAL HEALING AND DREAMS

It is to the regularity or mechanical uniformity of the working of our organism that Dr. Sigmund Freud of Vienna and his disciples trust in their rôle of Spiritual Healers through psycho-analysis. Their procedure is by analysis conducted either by skilful questioning or by the use of significant words, to lay bare gradually and surely the hidden links by which undesirable ideas and feelings are so held together as to produce a morbid state of consciousness. The subject-matter that is sought after may lie latent in waking consciousness, or may disclose itself in dreams. Dr. Freud has himself told us [1] how he came to turn his attention to the phenomena of dreams. He had for some time been engaged in a practical investigation of the various classes of phobias, of delusions and *idées fixes*, when it occurred to him that light might be thrown on his system of psycho-therapy from the dominion of dreams. "Phobias and fixed ideas are related," he observed, "to normal consciousness as are dreams to waking consciousness. A practical interest compels us to ascertain the origin and mode of development of these psycho-pathical ideas, since experience shows that the discovery of the uncon-

[1] *Über den Traum* in *Grenzfragen des Nerven- und Seelenlebens*, 1901, No. 8.

scious paths of association along which the morbid ideas accompany the general content of the mind leads to a mastery over the ideas which before were out of reach of all control."

Dr. Freud's analysis of dream-procedure is something of this sort. When we wake in the morning we sometimes remember our dreams, and these for the most part are dramatic representations of actions which in waking hours we should never perform, or of a series of grotesque, meaningless and incongruous actions which, so far as we can see, have no connection with the train of our waking thoughts and conduct. But, Dr. Freud contends, this disconnection is apparent only, for a patient inquiry into previous waking experiences will bring to light a series of emotional complexes, often inhibited complexes, which have afforded the raw material for the dream. And it is particularly unfulfilled desires or inhibited volitions which are largely responsible for the absurdities revealed in the dream. The contradictions, insults and ridicule of which we are victims when awake, are transmuted into absurdities when we dream. What, for example, is ordinarily regarded as a relation of cause and effect becomes in dreams the change of the one into the other, and conversely logical connection in waking consciousness becomes proximity in space or time when we dream.

The process, then, may be thus described summarily. Our thoughts, feelings and volitions when awake are the raw material out of which dreams are spun, and the immediate cause of the dream may be always found in some experience of the day

N

before the dream happens. This psychical complex as used may be called the "dream-thought." The mind "sub-consciously" works on this material, and in quite illogical manner weaves out of it something different in emphasis and proportion of parts from what happened when the subject was awake. This process may be called the "dream-work." Then comes what we remember of our dream when we wake, and this Freud calls the "dream-content." On this he sets to work so that he may translate it back into its original "dream-thought," and this work he calls "dream-analysis." Finally, he is able, as the result of his analysis, to point to the dreamer the precise spot where some psychical abnormality may have been at work, and so drag it out of its hiding-place in the "sub-conscious," and by putting it in the full light of consciousness, rob it of all its secret and unsuspected malefic influence.

What is true of troubles disclosed in dreams, is also true of troubles which lie beneath the surface of waking consciousness. The nature of the trouble is the same in both cases, and the remedy is the same. In the complex mechanism of that one and undivided concrete living thing we call a man, forces are at work which lie beneath the threshold of consciousness. Wrong modes of thought, wrong in the sense that they do not make for well-being, and are, therefore, it may be supposed, not in accord with Reality, are entertained all unknown to the consciousness of the subject. Thus I may fancy that I am going to be worsted in a parliamentary debate, or that I am suffering from cancer, or that I shall die in the workhouse, or that I am hated by my neighbour, or that I have committed the unpardonable sin, and even though I have sufficient power of reason to see that all such thoughts are delusions, yet I may not possess sufficient willpower to banish their reflexes in my psychical dispositions. Hence there arises a general pessimistic feeling, which envelops like a pall my whole waking self. The consequence of this morbid psychosis is that Life, which normally would pour its cleansing and invigorating streams through me, finds its road blocked, and can only get through in driblets. From this again result illnesses of many sorts, which form the staple occupation of the medical profession, but are in reality symptoms only of a bad state of the Soul. The psychologist, therefore, who, like Dr. Freud, can diagnose from the symptoms of the body their causes in the soul, and can then compel his patient to set to work to counteract his suppressed hallucinations, or dissolve his *idées fixes*, or dismiss his phobia, is in reality applying a spiritual power to a disease which, beginning in the patient's spirit, has infected his whole mechanism of living-body. And this is a mode of Spiritual Healing based on exact and verifiable knowledge of the process by which health degenerates into ill-health.

These considerations will, perhaps, enable us to answer somewhat more definitely the question suggested above as to the nature of "incubation" as practised in the temples of Asklepios. On Greek soil "incubation" took place, however, not only in the temples, but also at graves and holy wells. It may well be, as has been insisted on, that the temple-sleep in Greece is to be traced to Egypt as its origin,[1] and that the sacred sleep by the grave-side or at the holy well was autochthonous, as in other countries. But the distinction can be made too clear-cut for facts, seeing that a holy well was, as a rule to be found in every temple,[2] and that the temple, moreover, of a chthonian god of healing and divination was not infrequently erected over the burying-place of the god who, at an earlier stage, had been thought of as a "hero." A few examples of the practice of incubation may help us to understand better the ground out of which Spiritual Healing springs.

Plutarch [3] tells the following story of the oracular temple of Mopsus, a seer who became a hero and a god and was worshipped by the Cilicians as an incarnation of Apollo of Claros. The Governor of Cilicia, at the time of the story, was of a sceptical turn of mind, and a friend of Epicureans. On one occasion he sent to the oracle a freedman with a sealed tablet containing a question which was known to nobody. The messenger, according to custom, spent the night in the temple, and had the following dream. A man of beauteous form appeared to him, and called out simply "A black

<hr />

[1] As by O. Stoll, *Suggestion und Hypnotismus,* 1904, p. 311.

[2] *E. g.* at Epidauros, Kos, Oropos, the Athenian Asklepieion, Delphi. So Lourdes and St. Anne de Beaupré have their holy wells ; so also has Rome in the Fontana di Trevi, and Brittany in the spring of St. Morand. Philostratos (*Vita Apoll.* ii. 37) says : " I could mention many oracles, held in repute by Greeks and barbarians alike, where the priest utters his responses from the tripod after imbibing water and not wine," and this after saying a little before that, "as a faculty of divination that of dreams is the divinest and most god-like of human faculties."

[3] *De defectu oraculorum,* c. 45.

one," and then disappeared. This seemed extraordinary, and nobody could make anything out of it, but when the Governor heard it he was terrified, and fell to the ground in prayer, and then opening the tablet he showed the question written in it, which was: "Shall I sacrifice to thee a white or a black ox?" Upon this the Epicureans were perplexed, and the Governor made the sacrifice and ever afterwards held Mopsus in honour. The story, it is right to add, may be explained away as an invention or a legend, or accounted for by coincidence, suggestion, or fraud, or actual inspiration, according to our taste.

Pausanias again tells us [1] that in his time there existed a temple of Ino in Lacedæmon where men went to sleep in order, through dreams sent by the goddess, to learn their future.

At the grave of Orpheus at Olympus once a herdsman rested at midday. He fell asleep and began to sing with loud voice the songs of Orpheus, so that all the shepherds and peasants in the neighbourhood came to listen. In consequence of the crowding together of these, the pillars were overthrown on which lay the urns containing the bones of Orpheus, and as a punishment the oracle decreed that the State should be laid waste by an inundation.[2] The nature of the story is familiar enough, but the only point which concerns us is the natural way in which, when the story was formed, the incident of the dream-sleep was introduced.

Eusebius tells us that in Cilicia Constantine the Great had a temple destroyed in which a god, whom thousands honoured as their Saviour and

[1] *Lakonia*, c. 26.   [2] Pausanias, *Bœotia*, c. 30.

Physician, was wont to appear to sleepers and to heal their sicknesses.[1] And Pausanias tells us [2] of a house, behind the public square of Phlius, which the inhabitants called the house of the Diviner. Once Amphiaraos spent a night in this house, and from that time onwards he himself practised divination.

Before the altar of the Græco-Egyptian god, Serapis, the generals of Alexander the Great slept for many nights during his last illness. In the great temple of Amphiaraos at Oropus were altars to the healing gods Apollo, Athene and Heracles. Visitors in search of health would fast three days from wine and one day from food, and then sleep on the fleece of a ram sacrificed to the deity. So famous did this temple become that at one time it is said to have ruined all the Asclepieia in Bœotia.[3]

Æschylus tells us (in Pausanias) [4] that in his youth, when once he fell asleep at night in the hut of a vineyard, Bacchus appeared to him and bade him write a tragedy. This he proceeded to do the next day. Again, in the first Messenian war the hero, Aristodemos, who had been already upset by various portents, dreamed that his death was at hand, and this caused him to kill himself in despair.[5]

Strabo [6] tells us that healings took place at the temple of Serapis at Kanopus, and that "the most eminent men believe in it and sleep there for themselves or for others."

In these and the innumerable stories of dreams

[1] *De vita Constantini,* iii. 56.   [2] *Korinthia,* 13.
[3] See Mary Hamilton, *Incubation,* 1906, p. 80 ff.
[4] *Attika,* 21.   [5] *Messenia,* 13.
[6] *Geographica,* xvii. 1, 17.

which antiquity has handed down to us, we see a sharp line of distinction drawn between the consciousness of ordinary waking life, and that of sleep, by which the latter was regarded as the condition precedent for inspiration by some deity. Prof. Freud professes to have abolished this distinction by analyzing the contents of the dream consciousness into two elements, one supplied by the waking consciousness of the day preceding the dream, which acts as the stimulus, and one, experience that is past and stored up in memory. He does not, however, exclude and cannot exclude the possibility that these latent materials may be used and set in motion by the agency of living spirits, or by the transcendental Subject. And until this is done, to exclude the supernormal character of revelations given in dreams is illegitimate. In spite of all that modern science has done to explain the mechanism of mind, there still remains open the possibility, not to say the probability, that the folk-mind was, as usual, correct in its judgment that another aspect of Reality is opened to us in the dream-condition than that which meets us when we are, as we say, awake. Indeed, there is no antecedent improbability in the suggestion that the seeing of "ghosts" in broad daylight may be due to a momentary falling asleep without knowing it, so that for the moment a different order of existence impinges on our mind. And if this be a tolerable hypothesis, it is not difficult to see that the same power which thus gives second-sight may similarly, in favourable conditions, so stimulate the Life in us as to give for weakness health.

It is not, of course, to be supposed that Spiritual

Healing was the chief method of treatment in ancient Greece, for the *Corpus Hippocraticum* testifies to the existence of what Prof. Gomperz describes as a "not merely incomparable but no less than unique positive or rational science." But apparently in accordance with a well-known law, when science showed itself unprogressive, the Life-impulse burst its fetters, and used, as is customary, the "vulgar" as its readiest instruments. Somewhere about the end of the fifth century B.C., incubation or divination proceeded to supplement rational medicine more extensively. "The worship of Asklepios was introduced into Athens 426 B.C., and he henceforth became more widely known and more highly honoured, finally developing into Zeus-Asklepios, the Saviour κατ' ἐξοχήν of Greek popular religion, surviving all his fellow deities till we get a final glimpse of him about A.D. 450, when the philosopher Domninus, a Jew by faith, incubated in his temple and ate pork at his behest, a century after the legalisation of Christianity." From the "vulgar" this wave of Spiritual Healing spread to the cultured, and from them to the medical men in precisely the same way that it has done in our days among ourselves. The progress of this wave may be described in the words of Mr. E. T. Withington in the supplementary chapter written by him for the essay of Mr. W. H. S. Jones on *Malaria and Greek History*. On page 155 he says: "The malaria theory also helps to explain a remarkable development in the history of Greek religion. In the sixth century there had been a partial revival of the old Pelasgic worship, but the cult of the chthonian god of healing was kept in the background for some time longer by the prestige of the secular guild of the Asclepiadæ. This derived its name from Homeric sources, took the Homeric view of Asclepius, was Olympian in worship and rationalistic in practice. But just as ' the fear and sense of sin produced especially by the calamities of the sixth century ' caused a re-emergence of Pelasgian Orphism, purification, Dionysus-Zagreus worship, etc., so the spread of malaria seems to have brought forward once more the ancient Minyan earth-spirit with his therapeutic dream-oracle, which received thenceforward higher and higher recognition, till Zeus-Asclepius, Σωτὴρ τῶν ὅλων, seemed at one time a possible rival of the Saviour God of Christianity."

The only comment this passage requires is that rational medical science is by itself insufficient to satisfy the therapeutic requirements of even rational men, unless it has in some degree a cordial understanding and appreciation of the latent powers of the spiritual in man.

Before dismissing this subject one or two other examples of incubation may be referred to in order to show from the widespread character of the practice the probability that it rests on some ground of reason, however unmediated or unexplored that ground may have been.

In the Province of Madras a yearly festival is held in honour of the goddess Draupati, at which the ceremony of walking through fire forms a principal feature. Those about to take part in the ceremony prepared themselves for it several days before by bathing, fasting and sleeping in the temple of the goddess.[1] It is said that the Man-

[1] Stoll, *Suggestion und Hypnotismus*, 1904, p. 72.

darins of Amoy, when in perplexity about some judicial decision they were to give, would spend the night in the temple of the local god so as to get in dream the illumination they felt themselves in need of.[1] Whether the practice, however, still obtains seems to be somewhat doubtful. But Perham tells us that the Dyaks of North Borneo would spend one or several nights on a mountain-height so as to induce some beneficent spirit to bestow on them some power or honour they desired, or to set them free from some stubborn ailment by which they were afflicted.[2] In Eastern Australia a man obtained magical powers by sleeping on the grave of a newly-buried corpse.[3] In Guatemala an expression for a magician is the "Producer of the Sleep."[4] In Honduras, under the Spanish name of Nagual, was found a practice by which a man would sleep in the desert, or on a mountain, or by a river, and seek that his protecting god would come to him and make a compact to further his interests throughout his life.

Iamblichus tells us that the Babylonian women were in the habit of going into the temple of the goddess Zarpanit, the wife of Marduk, to sleep and dream. Their dreams were then interpreted by one of the seers whose special work it was to interpret dreams.[5]

Herodotus says of certain African savages : "The Nasamones go to the tombs of their ancestors, and after praying lie down to sleep, and whatever dream they have they make use of it."

---

[1] Stoll, *Suggestion und Hypnotismus*, 1904, p. 51.
[2] *Ibid.*, p. 99.   [3] *Ibid.*, p. 113.
[4] *Ibid.*, p. 169.   [5] *Ibid.*, p. 207.

In Africa again, according to Nachtigal, the ruler of the district of Tarti would, on New Year's Night, sleep in a hut erected for the purpose by the seaside. The dreams which then came to him were regarded as visions which possessed indubitable importance for the good of his district.[1] So in Madagascar the natives carried about with them a fetish which they called Aulis, and its possessor held conversations with this tutelary god, and sought his advice by means of dreams which came in holy sleep.[2]

It may seem a descent to bathos when we find a degenerate form of this religiously-minded incubation in the superstitious practice of some modern gamblers, who will dream of certain numbers and then put their dream to the test at the gaming-table.[3]

In all these cases we are faced with an impulse which is of cardinal importance to the understanding of the subject of Spiritual Healing. We are now beyond the earlier prejudice of savants, which made them dismiss all stories of primitive belief as due to ignorance and superstition, and are disposed to discriminate between the permanent desire or purpose which sprang, and still springs, from the uniform needs and capacities of our common human nature, and the ignorant explanation, or misguided practice, or inadequate means adopted to attain that desire or purpose. The impulse to be discerned alike in the cases just cited is that which drives us out to ensue life and see good days directly without the limitations set by the mechan-

---

[1] O. Stoll, *ut supra*, p. 297.
[2] *Ibid.*, p. 280.   [3] *Ibid.*, p. 667.

ism of ordinary life and experience. To swallow pills, undergo massage, to fast and use prescribed exercises is to put oneself under the routine of medicine as practised by rule. But the free spirit of man is apt to rebel, and rightly rebels, against being made the passive object of social or professional machinery, and it will from time to time assert its autonomy by breaking out in contempt of all the slow and mechanical process of orthodox medicine, and will still seek to go to the fountainhead of healing waters by prayer, suggestion, contemplation, "solar self-culture," or whatever else may be the modern equivalent for ancient approach to the gods in dream, ecstasy, or hallucination generally. Nor are we at liberty to say that the machinery by which our lives are ordinarily governed is of such exclusive importance that we ought in its interests to bar out all attempts of Life to assert its powers independently of this machinery. It would be nearer to the truth of things to say that Life is constitutive of health and of all healthgiving measures, while orthodox medical praxis is regulative, and has as its function to determine only the general lines and the main direction in which Life and health are to be sought. The best physician, then, will be one who to his knowledge of medical practice adds a wise recognition of the fact that Life plays the leading part in securing and maintaining health. In this case, whatever the means his experience suggests to him as likely to be beneficial, he is in the proper sense of the word a Spiritual Healer.

CHAPTER IX

SUGGESTION is a word which has received great emphasis in the more recent study of the phenomena of one important class of illnesses, those connected more closely with the nervous system. Sometimes it stands for the whole sum of the actual stimuli, which the external world applies to our organs of sensation and perception, as with Dr. Otto Stoll in his work on *Suggestion und Hypnotismus in der Völkerspsychologie*. This use of the term, however, is so wide as in covering everything to be applicable to nothing in particular. Stoll himself is open, as he seems aware, to this criticism, since he refers to critics who object to such a use of the term *Suggestion* as he makes because it designates the whole of our psychical life. Accordingly he defines it as psychical pressure (psychischer Zwang). "This element of psychical pressure to which our processes of thought are subjected is the characteristic mark of all proceedings which we describe as suggestion. For the intrusion of a new idea into our world of thought determines and guides its direction in a way independent of the Will, that is, compulsorily; gives it for a period a certain one-sidedness of thought and judgment, which amounts sometimes to direct defect. Suggestibility to which in our modes of thought we all in some degree fall victims is, therefore, the strait-waistcoat of thought which governs all our conduct and forms our judgment of truth and falsehood, our views of good and evil, of beauty and ugliness, our feeling of love and hatred." [1]

Others give a less sweeping definition of suggestion. The school of Bernheim regards suggestion as "the communication of any proposition from one person (or persons) to another in such a way as to secure its acceptance with conviction, in the absence of adequate logical grounds for its acceptance." This does not differ from Stoll's except in the emphasis it lays on "the alogical production of conviction" as the essence of suggestion. But inasmuch as this note of non-logicality embraces all our prejudices, moral maxims, social customs and conventions, as well as all that we derive from our innate imitativeness and inveterate hero-worship and from such feelings as family love, patriotism, party-spirit and religious feelings and beliefs, suggestion still comes to cover the whole machinery of our work-a-day life. And when it occurs in the form of mass-suggestion, operating upon large bodies of people we have one of the most terrible and irresistible of the psychical forces by which men and women are driven. The Crusades, the processes against witches of the Middle Age and the two centuries after it, the Flagellants and the pilgrimages such as those directed to Lourdes in search of cure are familiar instances of the increased suggestibility of men in crowds.

Other authorities are content to define suggestion

[1] *Op. cit.*, p. 702.

as the process by which ideas are unconsciously
assimilated and without adequate motive; or, as
the deliberate alteration, by word or gesture, of
another's nervous system by which entrance is
afforded to the desired idea; or as a psychical act
which blocks up all association-tracks of the nervous
system other than the one suitable for the presented
idea; or as a moral impression which one person
exerts on another; or as the invasion of consciousness by an idea without criticism or opposition.
To all these definitions, or descriptions, two factors
are common, viz. the absence of all logical activity
and the passivity of the will. In other words, suggestibility and mental activity are in inverse ratio,
and, therefore, suggestibility in general, and for
the purpose of Spiritual Healing in particular, is
at its highest potency when the mind is most
completely passive and receptive.

Of this condition the most familiar example now-
a-days is afforded by hypnotism. Though hypnotism has been an abnormal condition of human consciousness sufficiently in evidence in nature- and
culture-peoples of all ages and countries, yet its
emergence as a method of scientifically applied
therapeutics does not date in theory before the days
of James Braid seventy years ago, and in practice
before the days of Liébeault, or his follower, H.
Bernheim, professor of medicine at Nancy, forty
or fifty years ago. At first doubt was felt as to
whether the physiological or the psychological
factor was paramount, but a general agreement has
now been come to that the former is subsidiary and
the latter the predominant partner. The early

theories of Mesmer according to which the cures he effected were ascribed to a "fluid" which was made effective by touch (he did not use mesmeric passes) have been generally abandoned and treated with a scorn they do not altogether deserve,[1] except in the case of the impostors who give public performances of it for the benefit of the credulous. Yet if "animal magnetism"[2] be described as a term of inexactitude, at all events there appears good reason for thinking that analogies exist between psychic radiation and the "field" of an electro-magnet. Moreover mesmerism and suggestion are both real forces, though they are different. "We may have suggestion without mesmerism, or mesmerism without suggestion; a pseudo-mesmerism may occur which really is only suggestion, and a pseudo-suggestion which really is only mesmerism; while a suggestive mesmerism, or mesmeric suggestion, may also be effected, in which the two are indivisibly combined." A correspondent to the *Journal of the Society for Psychical Research*, vol. ix. p. 55, April 1899, gives the following story to illustrate the reality of magnetic radiation and the power, apart from suggestion, which may be exercised by some people on others, or possibly by all

---

[1] Mesmer appears to have suffered the usual fate of men who are before their time, and his theories are only now beginning to receive due recognition. They are summarized in Appendix C.

[2] The least misleading term for the force which Mesmer made use of is the Oriental term Prâna, the cosmic Force which when it is become the organizing principle of an animated body we call Life. This Life is a radiating force, and it was to this that Mesmer gave the name of "animal magnetism," though he insisted that this and ordinary magnetism were distinct.

people in certain conditions. The authority is given vaguely as that of an English M.D., and the anonymity would rob the story of any claim to authority were it not that similar experiences are quite common. The Doctor had as patient a retired Major, previously in service in India. Conversation having turned on mesmerism and similar subjects, the Major asked the Doctor to take hold of his hand, whereupon the latter felt a strong vibration similar to that excited by an electric current. The Major then told the Doctor that he had always possessed this influence, and that it had served him well in his command of his men. He had, however, been deterred from using it by an incident which had occurred when, with her consent, he had once mesmerized his sister-in-law, and been frightened by its success. He placed in her hands an unopened letter, and bade her read its sealed contents. She held it unopened in her hands and read the contents, which were found to be correct when the letter was afterwards opened. Stoll relates a similar incident within his own experience, and ascribes it somewhat hastily to suggestion, or coincidence, which in neither of these two cases can be regarded as a true cause.

Dismissing now for the moment the vexed question of "mesmerism," we turn to the practice of hypnotism proper, which can be easily studied in the standard works of C. Lloyd Tuckey, J. Milne Bramwell, A. Forel, R. H. Vincent and A. Moll, and in the records of experiments made by Mr. Gurney, which may be found in Vol. IV of the *Proceedings of the Society for Psychical Research.*

o

And the first question which these authorities are called on to answer for us is: "What is hypnotism?" The term is due to Braid, who substituted it for "mesmerism," and also gave a subjective explanation of the phenomena in place of the previously accepted objective causality. As his experience of hypnotic conditions increased, he proposed to collect it all under another new term, that of "monoideism," which he chose for the purpose of insisting that the condition of the hypnotized patient was due to his being possessed by one dominant idea, or several dominant ideas. "It mattered little whether these had existed in the subject's mind previously, or were afterwards verbally suggested by the operator. The latter acted like an engineer, and called into action the forces in the subject's own organism, controlling and directing them in accordance with the laws which governed the action of the mind upon the body." The importance of this view will be seen later on. Braid also used a telling argument against the theory of a "vital fluid" when he urged that if hypnotism were not due to the distribution of nervous energy in the patient's own organism, then a preacher or author would expend in his work an amount of "magnetic power" proportionate to the number of his hearers or readers. And he further insisted that the mental element associated with the administration of drugs had been unduly neglected. Latterly, he abandoned his theory of involuntary monoideism and concentration of the attention as an adequate explanation of the phenomena, and preferred to use the phrase "double-consciousness."

To Braid, indeed, belongs the honour of laying the foundations of a scientific theory of hypnotism, and later inquirers have done no more than build on the foundations he laid, and to adorn their building with illustrative facts drawn from their own practice and from the spacious fields of ethnography.

One later school, that of Charcot, or that known as the Salpêtrière School, must be mentioned, if only to be dismissed. According to this school hypnosis was a morbid state; it was a neurosis to be found only in the hysterical; women were better subjects than men; it was of no therapeutic value, and belonged properly to the department of nosology. This view is now abandoned, and it was the Nancy School which gave it its death-blow. Its fundamental fallacy lay in the attempt to lay the whole operation at the door of the physical, and to ignore the proofs that Braid had accumulated of the power of suggestion as a mental act. In other words all forms of Spiritual Healing are ruled out in the Salpêtrière, while they are compatible with the doctrines held in general by the Nancy School.[1]

Of course no two authorities in any department of thought would be found in entire agreement on every detail of the system held by them in common. The Hegelian School, for example, embraces many varieties of thought, as does the Neo-Kantian, or the Pragmatist, or, in another direction, the Ritschlian. But none the less, certain broad

---

[1] See an article by Dr. J. Milne Bramwell in *Proc. of Psych. Research Society*, vol. xii. pp. 205-209, entitled, "What is Hypnotism?"

principles will hold more or less loosely together
those who start from a common world-view. In
this sense we may speak of authorities like Bernheim, Forel, Moll, and in our own country Milne
Bramwell and Lloyd Tuckey as of the Nancy
School in contradistinction to that of Charcot.
They all agree in placing the phenomena of hypnotism on the psychical side, and in regarding the
physical means used as subsidiary. Where they
differ is in the explanations they give of the way
in which the psychical works, or of the essential
nature of the psychosis itself.

For example, Dr. Milne Bramwell in the masterly
exposition of hypnotic theories given in his
Hypnotism, chap. xii, states Bernheim's theory
as embodying these points—

(1) Nothing differentiates natural and artificial
    sleep.
(2) Hypnotic phenomena are analogous to many
    normal acts of an automatic, involuntary
    and unconscious nature.
(3) An idea has a tendency to generate its
    actuality.
(4) In hypnosis the tendency to accept sugges-
    tions is somewhat increased by the action
    of suggestion itself. Such increased sug-
    gestibility, one of degree, not of kind, alone
    marks any difference between the hypnotic
    and the normal state.
(5) The result of suggestion in hypnosis is
    analogous to the result of suggestion in the
    normal state.

To this Bramwell objects that hypnotism and

sleep are not identical, because in hypnosis the dream material comes from the outside and not from inside as in sleep; because the dream material is richer in natural sleep than in the hypnotic; and because the hypnotized person tries to translate his hallucinations into actions in a manner that finds no parallel in ordinary sleep. On the main point Moll, Braid and Lloyd Tuckey are in agreement with Dr. Bramwell, and the last points out that ordinarily if you talk to a sleeping person you wake him, but you do not the hypnotized person.

To the second point Bramwell replies that as a matter of observed fact patients are not subject to the will of the operator in the sense that they behave like automatic machines moved from outside with no will of their own, and he gives a number of instances from his own practice of the operator's will being successfully resisted by the hypnotic subject.

The third point is shifted, and in its place there is put the observed fact that very often a waking suggestion will provoke its opposite in the normal state; hence we cannot argue from the phenomena of normal life where suggestion may or may not act successfully to hypnotic states where suggestion, as a matter of fact, does act with general success.

The fourth point is faulty as attributing in the normal condition too much efficacy to bare-handed suggestion and too little to the subject's psychoses.

To the fifth point Bramwell points out *in limine* that the analogy between the phenomena of suggestion in the waking state and those in the hypnotic breaks down on the observation that certain strong

exciting causes which produce violent reactions in
the waking state, such as hope, fear, faith and
religious excitement, are either unnecessary in the
case of hypnotic suggestion, or, as in the case of
fear, are distinctly hostile. He then dwells on the
following important differences which mark off the
hypnotic state from the state evoked by normal
suggestion. In the hypnotic state a wide range of
phenomena can be produced at any time and many
simultaneously; one phenomenon can be immediately
changed into its opposite; the hypnotic phenomena
can be terminated at will, or they can be adjourned;
the suggestion will be invariably responded to provided it does not conflict with the patient's moral
sense or his powers; similar stimuli produce
identical results; hypnotic suggestions are frequently successful when the patient has for years
shown himself refractory to the same suggestions
when made in his waking state; hypnotic suggestion tends to gain strength by repetition.

So far we have been discussing some of the
phenomena of hypnotism alone, and are at all
events on safe ground when we conclude that one
point on which all its representative practitioners
are agreed is that it is due to suggestion. We are
not, however, qualified as yet to say what suggestion in itself is. Sir Douglas Powell, in a Note
contributed as Appendix A to "A Report of
Clerical and Medical Committee of Inquiry into
Spiritual Faith and Mental Healing," adopts a
dictionary definition, and says that suggestion is
"the action of any idea in bringing another idea
to mind, either through the power of associa-

tion or by virtue of the natural connection of the ideas." This loan, however, from the obsolete associationist school of psychology will help us little since it omits the characteristic feature of suggestion as applied in ordinary hypnotic treatment. It gives the genus, but not the species. As with Dr. Otto Stoll the definition covers so much ground that it fits none. It is true that Sir Douglas proceeds to illustrate his definition by reference to the influence of suggestion in allaying abnormal excitement, or impeded functioning, or in producing some desired end. But we still miss the point of connection between a suggested idea, which as such is rather regulative of dynamism than itself dynamic, and the physical result which follows from the exercise of psychic activity. We must, therefore, look a little more closely at suggestion as practised in therapeutics.

The first point that strikes us is that the effect of suggestion in general varies with the subject. It is no constant force whose effects may be mathematically predicted. As with a telegram, the impression made on the receiver depends not only on the sensations stirred up in the auditory or optical nerve-complex, but also on the *meaning* of what is said. But the meaning of a word or series of words is even more of the nature of a mental construct than the "synthesis of apprehension" we call sensation, or the synthesis of perception. It is the reflex act of the mind on the stimulus supplied by the suggestion, and the force and range of the suggestion are determined by native or acquired habits of the whole psychical self. Hence as no two people

to whom suggestion is made possess the same rich-
ness of experience or general capacity, the response
to suggestion varies indefinitely. Moreover, the
driving force which connects the suggestion with
the result which follows from it is not in the suggestion at all, but in the psychical disposition of
the subject. Hence if the suggestion is *regulative*
of what the patient does, it is his own self which
is the *constitutive* factor of the result.

For example, a notice is published, we will suppose, in the morning papers to the effect that plague
has broken out in London and is spreading. This
suggests to one reader that her daughter must be
fetched away at once; to another, a medical man,
that he must hasten at once to the centre of the
outbreak; to another that he should study Dr.
Creighton's *History of Epidemics in Britain;* to
another that he should write to *The Times* to
denounce the culpable negligence of the Local
Government Board; and to a fifth that he should
pray for the extirpation of the disease. Or, to
borrow another illustration from Dr. Bramwell, it is
as when to three race-horses is applied the same
stimulus of spur, voice and whip. One will respond
to the full and win, a second will respond and then
flag, and the third bolts in the wrong direction.
So with different men to whom the same suggestion
is made. What actual response they will make
depends on the nature of the psychical organism
to which the suggestion comes. One man will
carry out the suggestion in the simplest and most
direct way. Another will meet it with hindering
and perverting suggestions from the hidden depths

of his own nature, while a third will stoutly meet
it with a "contrary suggestion." Dr. Lloyd
Tuckey, in his evidence before the Committee
referred to, spoke of healing by suggestion consisting in the evoking of "the power within ourselves,
but not of ourselves, which makes for health."
And Dr. B. M. Wright, in his evidence, said that
Spiritual Healing could not be differentiated from
healing by suggestion, and added that "the organism itself has the power to do the work, though
religious teaching and traditions may sink into the
sub-consciousness and again be called forth by suggestion." Dr. Wright also distinguished between
"Spiritual Healing," as depending on a belief in
the intervention of some force outside which is
invoked, and "Mental Healing," as resting on
forces in the patient's own organism. Dr. W. F.
Cobb also, in his evidence, made a similar distinction when he said that though the results of
Spiritual and Mental Healing might be apparently
identical, yet there was a fundamental difference,
seeing that in the former Christ was the direct
Healer through a human channel, while he implied
that the latter required no special influence from
the spiritual sphere. The Divine power to heal
was present and ever ready to act, but required
some focus through which to act before it could
become effective.

It is not easy to say what influence each of the
many simultaneous factors in hypnotism contri-
butes. That attention in some degree is necessary
appears from the fact that idiots, imbeciles and
those suffering from *idées fixes* (hysterics) are bad

subjects. Yet the attention which is negative is sufficient; abstraction, or reverie, or some quite obscure condition such as is supplied by the reminder of an earlier hypnosis will be effectual. The exclusive relation between operator and subject, which was once thought necessary to hypnosis and characteristic of it, has been made doubtful. Nor are the normal phenomena of suggestion in waking life, or of dream-consciousness able to account for the phenomena of hypnotism. More light, perhaps, is thrown on these latter by Mr. Myers's theory of the "subliminal self" already referred to, or by what Dr. W. B. Carpenter, as a physiologist, preferred to regard as "unconscious cerebration." The theory of a "secondary consciousness" functioning independently of the primary consciousness finds general favour, though many would shrink from carrying this consciousness so far as to establish a secondary personality. The cases described, however, in Sidis and Goodhart's *Multiple Personality* open up startling possibilities of our psychical life which have not yet received any satisfactory solution.

But of the value of hypnotism as a therapeutic agent in certain classes of cases there is no longer room for doubt. It is not a universal remedy, and is not directly curative in cases of "organic disease." But in cases of "functional" disorder, or in cases where the mind is a disturbing element, or sometimes where drugs are ineffective, its beneficial results are well known. Probably escape from the pressure of realism in philosophy and materialism in common life will issue in an increasing recourse to hypnotism in the earlier stages of illness, and in this case the preventive efficacy of hypnotism may be found to be more salutary even than its therapeutic.

It only remains, for our present purpose, to emphasize the facts (1) that suggestion, strictly speaking, is but the signal which starts into activity the Life-force in the material organism, just as a pistol-shot starts runners in races. When once started the direction it takes is determined by the total disposition of the organism itself, both physical and psychical; (2) that the cures effected by suggestion and subsequent hypnosis are not due directly to these agencies, but to the redintegrating activity of the Life itself; (3) that the general acceptance (after much opposition) by the medical faculty of hypnotism is an admission that man is more than an animated machine; he is that, but he is also the subject of a Force of Life which not only resides in him, but also acts on him and through him; (4) that the difficulty of explaining the *modus operandi* of hypnotic consciousness, as, *e. g.* in the power it shows in the measurement of time, is of the same character, and probably proceeds from the same root as the difficulty of explaining the interaction in general of mind and body, or even more of the ideal Ego and the empirical Ego. That startling cures are effected through hypnotism is certain. That even a greater field of therapeutics lies open, if not for hypnotism, at all events for waking suggestion, is probable. As to the explanation of how the process works, the history of human thought seems to bid us be content with saying,

"Ignoramus et ignorabimus," for no valid philosophic thought has yet carried us securely beyond
a methodological dualism.

It should now be clear that the Clerical and
Medical Committee referred to above have said
nothing in saying that "the physical results of what
is called ' Faith ' or ' Spiritual ' Healing do not
prove on investigation to be different from those
of Mental healing or healing by ' Suggestion,' " and
that they have completely steered clear of the facts
when they have contented themselves with saying
that "the term Suggestion is used in this Report as
meaning the application of any natural mental
process to the purpose of treatment."

We might suggest that attention be paid to the
judicious remarks of the well-known alienist, Dr.
James H. Hyslop, on this subject. Writing in
the *Quest* for October 1913 he pointed out that
suggestion was eagerly seized as a useful term of
explanation by those who wanted to rebut the super-
naturalism of the phenomena associated with the
activities of Mesmer. "From that time on," he
proceeds to say, "' suggestion ' has become a
universal solvent when a man wants to get out of
a difficulty. It was never, in fact, an explanation of
anything, and I doubt if any man, living or dead,
could tell exactly what he means by the term; but
it is very useful for throwing dust in the eyes of
the public. It names no known cause, and only
increases mystery instead of removing it. But it
keeps the public at bay, and that is its chief
function. As a means of frightening away false
ideas it is, and has been, useful; but as a means

of explanation it is absolutely worthless. It only represents a change of *venue* in trial of what the phenomena are, and the point of view from which they have to be studied. 'Suggestion' does not name any known cause, and until it does so it is no better than 'odylic force' or some supernatural agent, which, if it were a familiar one, might be a reasonable hypothesis. So far as explanation is concerned 'suggestion' is a subterfuge, though important for pointing out the group of facts that are possibly inconsistent with fluidic theories. But it leaves the whole mystery where it found it. It does not clear up any perplexity. It had and has only a use for encouraging the pretence of knowledge. It may silence ignorant believers in the supernormal, just as Dr. Johnson silenced the old fish-woman in Billingsgate by calling her an isosceles triangle. Ignorance could make no reply to that. In fact 'suggestion' is as supernormal a fact as telepathy or clairvoyance, judged from the standpoint of ordinary causation."

CHAPTER X

"MASS-SUGGESTION"

In Lord Morley's *Diderot* is the remark that "incredulity is sometimes the vice of a fool, and credulity the defect of a man of intelligence. The latter sees far into the immensity of the Possible; the former scarcely sees anything beyond the Actual." In no subject is there more danger, perhaps, of the student falling a victim to either stupidity or credulity than in that of Spiritual Healing. For it lies on the narrow ground which separates Life, Religion and Freedom on the one side from Machinery, Science and Necessity on the other, where it is easy to settle down on either side and to ignore the other. Credulity is no doubt an evil, but hardly greater than incredulity, and in the domain of Spiritual Healing there is much which now makes a thorough-going incredulity irrational.

For example, the power of Mass-suggestion is demonstrably enormous, and cases of it may be drawn from all quarters. We first will take two illustrative examples, one from Lourdes [1] and one

[1] We have already, in Chap. V, discussed the "Miracles" at Lourdes. Here we are concerned only with those circumstances of the pilgrimages which may be thought to apply in a forceful way to the sub-consciousness of the patients the *vis viva* of Mass-suggestion.

from Treves, and then support these by one or two less familiar cases.

On February 11, 1858, a peasant-girl, Bernadette Soubirous, saw Our Lady at the Grotto of Lourdes, for the first time, and the vision and its circumstances are thus described in an inscription cut on a marble tablet, which is erected near the Grotto, which runs—

Dates of the Eighteen apparitions
and words of the Blessed Virgin
in the year of grace 1858
In the hollow of the rock where her statue is now seen
the Blessed Virgin appeared to Bernadette Soubirous
Eighteen times.
The 11th and the 14th February ;
Each day with two exceptions, from February 18th till March 4th,
March 25th, April 7th, July 16th
The Blessed Virgin said to the child on February 18th
"Will you do the favour of coming here daily for a fortnight ?
I do not promise to make you happy
In this world, but in the next ;
I want many people to come."
The Virgin said to her during the fortnight :
"You will pray for sinners ; you will kiss the earth for sinners.
Penitence ! Penitence ! Penitence !
Go and tell the priests to cause a chapel to be built ;
I want people to come thither in procession.
Go and drink of the fountain and wash yourself in it.
Go and eat of that grass which is there."
On March 25th the Virgin said :
"I AM THE IMMACULATE CONCEPTION."

The visions soon became famous, and the dirty water of the Grotto a miraculous fountain. A stone-cutter, "one of whose eyes had been entirely destroyed," was the first person to be cured by it, and at the end of the appointed fortnight an enormous crowd had assembled. The wise officials of this world were disposed to imprison Bernadette, as their manner is, and on June 8 the police boarded up the Grotto. Two months later the Bishop of Tarbes appointed a Commission to investigate the miracle, and after a leisurely examination the Bishop decreed on January 18, 1860, as follows—

"We give sentence that Mary Immaculate, Mother of God, has really appeared to Bernadette Soubirous on February 11, 1858, and the following days, to the number of eighteen times, in the Grotto of Massabielle, near the town of Lourdes; that this apparition carries with it all the marks of truth, and that the faithful have good ground for believing it certain." The sanctity of Lourdes was afterwards affirmed by a Papal rescript.

It is calculated that about 600,000 pilgrims find their way every year to Lourdes, nearly all in search of health. August is naturally the busiest month at Lourdes, but all through the year the stream of pilgrims is incessant. Over the Grotto a church has been built with a crypt and a Church of the Rosary added. All the wealth of Catholic ceremonial, the whole "dazzling array of chandeliers, lamps, banners, statues, decorations the most varied," flags of all nations, music of all ages, processions and all the traditional knowledge and skill in suggestion of which the Catholic Church is possessed, are made to combine in instilling into the minds of the pilgrims the belief that they are going to be cured. And cured a large number are. Of these, according to Father Clarke, about two per cent. are ultimately classed as miraculous.

But quite apart from the ambiguity attaching to the word miraculous, it is becoming increasingly difficult to refer even striking cures, and cases which orthodox medicine may declare incurable, to the introduction of non-natural causation, such as the direct and, in the strict sense, "supernatural" intervention of Our Lady. Moreover, in Bernadette's revelations nothing was said of the institution of a curative procedure. This has been built up on precedents in Catholic lands, which find their prototype in classical times. What took place in the Asclepieia of Greece may be readily and safely conjectured from what takes place at Lourdes to-day. The names are changed and the place, but the underlying process is the same, the agency is the same, and the whole transaction starts from the same springs in our composite human nature. Enthusiasm is endemic, and a common faith grows in crowds whenever an adequate suggestion is forthcoming. The traditional piety of the people, stimulated by the apparitions and intensified by "mass-suggestion," is sufficient explanation of the cures that are effected. "These southern valleys," says Father Clarke, "are all of them remarkable for their Catholic spirit, and they have always kept their faith in spite of revolution and heresy." Need we look further than mass-suggestion falling on expectant and ardent spiritual life for the Spiritual Healing, be it on a large scale or a small, recorded in the *Annales de Lourdes?* There is no need or room for the miraculous in the ordinary sense of that ambiguous word.

At Treves,[1] the old Roman colony on the banks

---

[1] R. F. Clarke, *Pilgrimage to the Holy Coat of Treves,* 1892; E. A. Plater, *The Holy Coat of Treves,* 1891.

P

of the Moselle, we come across psychological phenomena resembling those of Lourdes. For there in
the Cathedral reposes the Holy Coat of Jesus
Christ, which was received from St. Helena—the
seamless robe mentioned by St. John, for which the
soldiers cast lots, of which mediæval legend reported
that "Christ's Holy Mother made for her Divine
Son while still a boy this seamless robe, and that
it not only did not grow old, but grew with His
growth, adapting itself to the form and size of His
sacred limbs." "This is, of course, possible," adds
Father Clarke, "for all things are possible with
God," though he does go on to say that it is
improbable.

For seven centuries Treves forgot all about its
treasure, but in 1196 it was taken out of hiding and
laid beneath the altar of St. Peter in the Cathedral.
In 1512 it was "exposed" at the prompted desire
of the Emperor Maximilian I. During the Thirty
Years' War its experiences were like those of the
Ark of the Covenant, but in 1759 it was taken back
to Treves, again six years later sent away, and
finally restored in 1810. Over a million pilgrims
visited it in 1844, and nearly two millions in 1891.
There was, however, on both occasions "the same
continual stream of pilgrims passing through the
church; the same perfect order and regularity; the
same edifying devotion on the part of the pilgrims;
the same wonderful graces flowing into the souls
of all who came thither; the same extraordinary
conversions of hardened sinners; the same miracles
worked on the bodies of the sick; the same impulse
given to the faith in all the country round; the same

oft-repeated calumnies on the part of the enemies of religion; the same present sense of God's grace and blessing on the part of all who took part in the spectacle." In short, to put Father Clarke's lyrical language into cold prose, there were all the phenomena of mass-suggestion, followed by the usual results.

But lest it be thought that orthodox Catholicism has any monopoly of cures by mass-suggestion, reference may be made to the cures and other miracles wrought at the tomb of the young Abbé François de Pâris, who died in 1727 and was buried in the cemetery of St. Médard. The Abbé had belonged to the Jansenists, and under Jesuit influence the cemetery was closed, and this police action gave rise to the sarcastic lines found by Voltaire on the cemetery wall—

> De par le Roi défense à Dieu
> De faire miracle en ce lieu.

Hume says of the strange occurrences : "There surely never was so great a number of miracles ascribed to one person, as those which were lately said to have been wrought in France upon the tomb of the Abbé Pâris. The curing of the sick, giving hearing to the deaf and sight to the blind, were everywhere talked of as the effect of the holy sepulchre. But what is more extraordinary, many of the miracles were immediately proved upon the spot before judges of unquestioned credit and distinction, in a learned age, and in the most eminent theatre that is now in the world." Among the cases of cure there are mentioned "incurable blindness, paralysis, dropsy and cancer." On the other hand, there were produced those cases of "hysterical paroxysms, fits of catalepsy, convulsions, hallucinations, prophesyings, visions, and the voluntary suffering of horrible bodily tortures," which have made famous the convulsionaries of St. Médard. This second class of phenomena is a useful reminder to us that suggestion may be as potent an influence on the side of the abnormal and undesirable as on that of the normal and beneficent. And the history of the "nature-peoples" and "culture-peoples" alike testifies to this fact. The Flagellants of the thirteenth and fourteenth centuries reflected the troubled state of social and political affairs at the time; they reappeared in succeeding centuries, chiefly among the lower ranks of Catholic piety, and from time to time find representatives at the great festivals of the Church. The "running-amok" of the Malays, resting though it may on an early ceremonial practice of tribes of Further India, is, however, in the form described by the phrase, the immediate product of mass-suggestion acting on unbalanced minds. The bloody orgies which distinguish the Feast of Hassan and Hussein as celebrated by the Persian colony in Constantinople, offer a terrible example of the potentialities for blood-lust, which can be let loose by suitable mass-suggestion.

Stoll relates in some detail [1] an extraordinary psychical epidemic which took place in South Brazil between 1872 and 1883, arising from an enthusiastic carpenter, who for some years had been known far

[1] *Suggestion und Hypnotismus*, 1904, p. 465 ff.

and wide as a Spiritual Healer. His wife was an epileptic, who learned gradually the art of bringing on a catalepsy at will and of inducing the hypnotic state. In this condition she acted as a clairvoyant, and announced the remedies which her husband's patients should use. Out of this grew, quite in keeping with the widespread connection of divination and healing, a practice of Bible-reading, which was concluded by the induction of the trance-condition, and the giving forth of prophetic utterances. Stretched on her bed in this state, "strange, slowly-spoken expressions, bombastic exhortations or prophecies came out of her mouth and filled the hearers with mysterious shuddering and reverential awe of one who seemed a higher being." Finally, the woman gave herself out as Christ and appointed apostles as He had done. The effect of her suggestions on numbers of people was so great that it led to bloodshed and the subsequent suppression of the movement by military violence. The account of this peculiar outbreak, as given by the Jesuit Father Ambros Schapp, is most instructive for those who want to understand the rise of propaganda such as that of Christian Science, or of pilgrimages in search of health to sacred spots, such as Lourdes in modern times, or the shrine of St. Thomas à Becket or our Lady of Walsingham in the Middle Age.

What an effective part suggestion may play in the healing of disease, and especially "mass-suggestion," may be easily seen in the history of Tarantism in South Italy. The bite of the tarantula is poisonous, but apparently not more so than

the sting of a wasp. It was for long considered
to be the cause of the disease named after the spider,
tarantism, a belief which science has exploded.
"According to traditional accounts, the first symptom of this disorder was usually a state of depres-
sion and lethargy. From this the sufferer could
only be roused by music, which excited an over-
powering desire to dance until the performer fell to
the ground bathed in profuse perspiration, when
the cure, at all events for the time, was supposed
to be effected. This mania attacked both men and
women, young and old alike, women being more
susceptible than men. It was also considered to be
highly infectious, and to spread rapidly from person
to person until whole areas were affected." [1] It is
now generally admitted that the phenomena of
tarantism are not to be ascribed to any poisonous
bite, but to the suggestive power of folk-belief,
which gives rise to an auto-suggestive terror, which
in its turn will sometimes produce a catalepsy.
The tarantula-dance is a means to this end, [2] and
serves at the same time to bring about a condition
in which belief in the cure is rendered possible.
From the antiquity and wide diffusion of music and
dancing as means of producing ecstasy, we may
fairly suspect that the spider of Taranto in Apulia
is but an object on whom an accident of history
has fastened this ancient ceremonial.

To mass-suggestion also may be assigned that

---

[1] *Encyc. Brit.*, xi. edn. vol. xxvi. p. 416, s. v.

[2] We should compare with this the well-known passage in
which Rohde (*Psyche*, p. 302 f.) describes the effects of the
Dionysiac dance.

stubborn root of "superstition" which even the most
modern man finds it difficult to extirpate wholly.
The uneasy feeling which follows the spilling of
salt, sitting down thirteen at table, passing under
a ladder, finding knives crossed, or speaking of
good fortune; the belief in amulets, in lucky days,
in relics, in holy wells, in indulgenced devotions,
rests on the uncritical and traditional beliefs of the
many around us, from which we are unable or un-
willing to shake ourselves free. "Even the pilgrimages made by pious people down to modern times
to holy places, for the purpose of securing for
themselves or others healing from some disease, are
at bottom nothing else but a form of the old
Incubation ; and their suggestive effect rests on the
same principle, although no doubt it expresses itself
for the most part as the auto-suggestion of the
waking state."

As an example of mass-suggestion asserting itself
through auto-suggestion and showing its power
through such alterations of the vascular system as
tumours, wounds and stigmata, the case of Anna
Katharina Emmerich may be cited.[1] She was born
of peasant-stock in 1778, became a nun in 1802 and
died in 1824. Enamoured of suffering through
continual meditation on the wounds of the
Redeemer, she gradually fell a victim to hysteria,
epilepsy and convulsions, and showed traces of
clairvoyant powers, prophetic gifts and a longing
for therapeutic miracles. In addition to this the
stigmata of Jesus Christ began to appear in her.
"On the back of the hands, on the feet, in the palm

[1] Otto Stoll, *Suggestion und Hypnotismus*, 1904, p. 521 ff.

of the hands and in the soles of the feet appeared wounds, those on the back of the hands and the upper part of the feet being larger than those in the palms and soles. On these wounds lay a crust of blood as thin as paper, the skin near the wounds was stained with blood, and the wounds were painful when touched." The nun was kept under close and skilful medical observation, and no doubt exists that she was not an impostor, and that her case was not got up by the clergy for their own purpose. The explanation is that certain receptive natures have the power of reacting powerfully on suitable stimuli, especially, as in the case before us, on objective suffering. So far may this reaction be carried, that not only is the pain of the other actually felt, but vascular changes are effected in the organism of the sympathetic observer. In consequence, as medical science has crystallized the receptiveness which issues in imitative sounds and actions as *echolalia* and *echopraxia*, so it would call the morbid state of Anna Emmerich *echopathia*.

The importance of this "irritability" for the understanding of Spiritual Healing, and indeed for its further progress, can hardly be over-estimated. For if a mass-suggestion can be obtained, in accordance with which the psychical air around us is full of germs carrying with them ideas which tell us that health is normal, and what ought to be, and that disease is abnormal and what ought not to be, we should then find it easy to suggest, whether to ourselves or to others, images of healthy and robust humanity by which the necessary vascular changes might be produced in those who were sufficiently

receptive of them. And then we might discover
that after all health was as contagious as disease,
and succeed finally in making it endemic to humanity. This would be a triumph indeed for Spiritual
Healing.

If anybody is disposed to object to this dream
that it can be never more than a dream because we
know now so much of the human organism that
we can say positively what is possible and what is
not possible, he may be invited to consider the case
quoted expressly in answer to a similar objection in
Vol. IX of the *Proceedings of the Psychical Research Society.* According to the report of this
case made by the medical man himself, a Mr. J. W.
Teale of Scarborough, presented on February 26,
1875, to the Clinical Society of London, the case
of a lady under his care who, on September 5, 1874,
had fallen from her horse and broken her ribs; she
maintained for seven consecutive weeks a temperature never found less than 108 degrees; and one
which on four several days was of 122 degrees.[1]
In spite of this unheard of condition the patient
recovered and the medical press jeered. Mr. Teale,
however, produced his proofs. "Seven thermo-
meters had been used for the observation. Three
of these were made specially for the occasion. Four
were sent to be tested at Kew, and found correct
within a tenth of a degree. Each thermometer was
inspected by two or three trustworthy witnesses
before and after each observation, and the results

---

[1] On November 12, at 10.10 p.m., her temperature was
registered at 113·6 degrees ; on November 13, at 4 a.m., 122
degrees, and on the same day at 10 a.m., 114·3 degrees.

were at once recorded in writing. No hot-water bottles were near the axillæ. The temperature was taken in two and sometimes three parts of the body simultaneously. Each thermometer, after having been shaken down to normal, was changed in position, and readings again compared, to eliminate any local accident or fraud. Finally, these elaborate observations were continued daily for ten weeks. And thus "in spite," as the *Lancet* said, "of the widespread consternation at such a revolution of (previous) notions, yet it was impossible to question the accuracy of the record." [1]

The purpose of the S.P.R. in quoting this peculiar case was to illustrate the duty of taking particular care in testing psychical phenomena by the extreme care taken by physical or physiological science to test the cases brought before it. But another deduction may be made from it, and that is the danger of letting ourselves suppose that the observations of science are sufficient to establish any ultimate principle. The induction of observed facts may be as large as you please, and may justify you in establishing a working hypothesis, but can never constitute a principle of Reality. At any moment our hypothesis may be shown to be partial by the emergence of some new fact thrown up in the indeterminate activity of Life. And where this Life is working through so highly developed an organism as that of man, it should not be disconcerting to us if the surprises it gives us are greater here than elsewhere. But, indeed, the phenomena of healing by mass-suggestion are so widespread in space and time that they ought not now-a-days to strike anybody as incredible. And as Wieland has said : "Perhaps it is exactly the greatest man of science who least ventures to declare anything impossible which does not obviously belong to the class of four-angled triangles."

And in the same sense Sir Clifford Allbutt writes [1] that "no limb, no viscus is so far a vessel of dishonour as to be wholly outside the renewals of the spirit." And Sir Henry Morris, writing as a champion of medical science, says : "In faith-healing the suggestion is that cure will be worked by spiritual or Divine power, especially if this power be appealed to at some particular place, such as a sanctuary, the foot of an idol, a fountain, or pool of water, the resting-place of some sacred relic, such as the bones of a saint, or it may be in presence of the Eucharistic procession, or during High Mass, or the administration of the Holy Sacrament. . . . This Divine power or energy is supposed to act by neutralizing or overcoming sickness, disease and the ill consequences of accident. The faith-healer does not doubt the reality of matter or of disease, but believes that he can draw upon a spiritual force to subdue or annihilate an existing evil." [2]

Finally, a striking instance of the futility of trying to limit the possible by the known is afforded by the present King's story of the vision of the *Flying Dutchman* when he was in the Navy.

When in 1881 the *Bacchante* was being repaired for an injured rudder, the King and his brother

[1] *British Medical Journal,* June 18, 1910, p. 1483.
[2] *Ibid.,* p. 1458.

were transferred to the *Inconstant*, in which vessel they remained from July 8 to August 2. It was in the *Inconstant*, during the passage from Melbourne to Sydney, that the incident of the *Flying Dutchman*, described as follows in the Princes' journal, took place on July 11—

"At 4 a.m. the *Flying Dutchman* crossed our bows. A strange red light as of a phantom ship all aglow, in the midst of which light the masts, spars and sails of a brig 200 yards distant stood out in strong relief as she came up on the port bow. The look-out man on the forecastle reported her as close on the port bow, where also the officer of the watch from the bridge clearly saw her, as did also the quarter-deck midshipman. . . . Thirteen persons altogether saw her, but whether it was *Van Diemen* or the *Flying Dutchman*, or who else, must remain unknown. . . . At 10.45 a.m. the ordinary seaman who had reported the *Flying Dutchman* fell from the foretopmast crosstrees on to the topgallant forecastle and was smashed to atoms."[1]

It is also worth noting that the Committee appointed by the Dialectical Society in 1873 reported that they were satisfied that "there is a force capable of moving heavy bodies without material contact, and which force is in some unknown manner dependent upon the presence of human beings."

[1] *Times*, July 4, 1914, p. 9.

CHAPTER XI

WE have now taken as extensive a view of the field of Spiritual Healing as is possible within the limits set to the present volume. But though the investigation has been necessarily of a general character, so that the greater part of the story still remains untold, yet the writer hopes that he has not omitted any feature whose loss would vitiate the truth which the Spiritual Healer holds in trust. If this be so, all that remains is to draw out of the material before us its permanent factors, and to make a few tentative suggestions in our turn to all who are interested in our subject.

1. The first fact which strikes us is the ubiquity of Spiritual Healing in some form or other. The earliest records as well as the latest tell of it; it is not confined to any grade of culture, for "culture-peoples" as well as "nature-peoples" are familiar with it. No doubt, it may be urged, the former show it, and Lourdes, Christian Science, holy wells and Bethshan can be adduced as lamentable examples of superstitious survivals of folk-credulity in a cultured age. But in reply to this we may surely retort that the objection rests on an unproved contempt for the folk-mind. It may be true that the

folk describe and the scientists explain, but this does not necessarily mean that the description is proved false by the explanation. The folk-mind may not be analytical, or critical, and may give in its haste premature or one-sided explanations which a more reflective age finds insufficient. And for all that the activity of the folk-mind may be a valid part of human culture. Because it has been improved on it does not follow that it has been destroyed, unless we are to say that when a lower thing has been subsumed by a higher, the lower has ceased to be. The burden of proof, anyway, of the uselessness for science of the pronouncements of the folk-mind rests on their accuser, not on their counsel. Perhaps, then, we may say that while the folk-mind is apt to let its feelings run away with its judgment, yet those feelings are not empty or negligible, but do witness to certain factors in human nature which different stages of culture may appraise, or use differently, without being able to dispense with them altogether.

2. The second fact which is inevitable is the general identity of the means employed in every stage of culture by practitioners of the art of Spiritual Healing. Incubation as a means of securing help through dreams is witnessed to generally. The laying on of hands, or stroking, or the making of passes, or rubbing in various forms is equally familiar. The use of objects to which sanctity for some reason is supposed to attach is common everywhere. So, too, is the recitation of a "word of power," and the belief in the special powers of certain persons, shamans, medicine-men, priests

or priestesses. Holy wells still are thought to
retain their healing powers, and holy places are
resorted to in the same way and for the same
purpose as similar holy places were three thousand
years ago.

The persistency of these habits of thought may
no doubt be interpreted in either of two ways. The
exclusive lover of right reason will see in them the
incorrigible inability of the mass of men to order
their lives strictly by abstract thought, and he will
lament the stubborn refusal of feeling to submit
itself to Reason. On the other hand, the more
philosophic mind, remembering that the claim of
Reason to exclusive jurisdiction is itself a superstition, will see in the very persistency of the means
of healing here in question a testimony to something
corresponding to them in the world of Reality. He
may even be disposed to put in the evidence of
great religious teachers as to the power of faith
over reason, when this latter is taken in the narrower
sense. And as faith, or trust, is faith or trust in
some objective reality, he will venture to affirm the
high probability of this age-long faith being but the
instinctive recognition by the untutored human
mind of *something* in its universe which will
operate, if it can only be got hold of, to remove
pain and sickness and disease in general. In presence of the general prevalence of this belief in
savage, barbarous and civilized peoples alike we
submit that the burden of proving its falsity rests
on those who oppugn it, not on those who defend
it, especially when the evidence for the success of
the belief when acted on is shown to be not only

copious, but self-coherent and capable of rational explanation.

3. A third point which seems to be particularly worthy of attention is the prevalence of the belief in the agency of Spirit, or spirits. This is not confined to one age or place or stage of culture, but is common to all. For whether we look at the suppliants of Æsculapius, or those who sought relief at the hands of Jesus Christ, or who have recourse to the séance-room, or go on pilgrimage to Lourdes or Treves, the appeal is made to Spirit to give relief to incarnate spirits from disorders which are assigned in many cases to the sinister working of other spirits. This latter clause has a less general reference than it would have had four hundred years ago, but until the Renaissance it found few men bold enough to deny it. The reason why it is no longer in evidence is the spread of the scientific attitude of mind, an attitude which is directed more towards the machinery of things than to their origin in Life, and hence is tempted to emphasize the material- or form-side as best able to account for phenomena. Yet the more learning which Bacon desiderated leads from this one-sided view to the larger view which sees the creative cause of all motion in Spirit, and attributes healing, therefore, not to a more skilful collocation of atoms, or mere adjustment of the organism to its environment, but in the letting loose by Spirit of life-giving forces which sweep before them the evils of sickness and disease. And many not irrational people will say that from the positing of Spirit to its differentiation into living centres is but a short and perhaps

a necessary step. Spirit seems to imply those finite centres which we call spirits and distinguish for our convenience into good and evil.[1]

It seems the more necessary to urge the relevancy of the appeal to the activity of spirits not in physical flesh on spirits like ourselves which are at present in physical flesh, because of the discredit into which it has fallen. For unless we are to assume that the whole history of mankind is but a record of helpless superstition we are bound to say how we account for the persistency of the belief in the present activity of excarnate spirits. It is easy to say that primitive man projected his own self-consciousness on Nature around him and so erected the doctrine of Animism. But this view implies illegitimately that primitive man was not justified in doing this, which is precisely the point requiring to be proved. Besides, no explanation is given of the fact that it is not primitive man alone who is guilty, but that all men in all stages do in some degree the same thing. The more rational conclusion is that the persistency of the belief in spirits is the reflection in consciousness of a corresponding existence in reality; in other words, man believes in spirits because spirits exist. Of course, in taking up this position we are open to the warning that such a belief is the fertile mother of credulity, hasty judgments, unwholesome fears, and the gravest obstacle we know to the progress of a rational view of the

---

[1] *Cf.* McTaggart : " The Absolute must be differentiated into persons, because no other differentiations have vitality to stand against a perfect unity, and because a unity which was undifferentiated could not exist." *Studies in Hegelian Cosmology,* 1901, p. 17.

Q

world. This is quite true, and yet is no argument against the activity of spirits, but only a much needed warning against letting our feelings get the mastery over our reason.

This is not the place to argue over again the controversy which has raged over Animism. It is enough to say that in so far as this doctrine is taken to mean the existence of a sort of "mannikin" abiding as the subject of our feelings, volitions and thoughts but distinct from them, this is not the position advocated here. What does seem required by a metaphysic which shall in its theory of Being make due allowance for the phenomena of Spiritual Healing, is that it shall not only regard all that is real as mind, but regard Reality as an organization of selves which interact on each other. That is to say, our metaphysic will not be content with a Universe in which the Reality is the hidden "Force" and the phenomenal world its (comparatively) unreal appearance, but will on the contrary treat both Life and its appearances as aspects of Reality, and thus accept the Universe as a pluralistic Reality with an idealistic unity. This is what we may suspect Mrs. Eddy would have wished to say had she known how to say it. What she seems to have said and what many are saying with her is that if we can slough off our fond belief in the reality of phenomena, and, ignoring them, get behind them to the one living Reality that is called God, we shall be able to seat ourselves as assessors to His throne, and, like Phœbus Apollo, turn the rays of healing power whither we will. This current belief we hold to be at once bad, both as a metaphysic and as a religion, and submit that on the contrary a belief in spirits and their activity is sane and rational. What the nature of excarnate spirits may be like, or what is the mode of their acting, is for the most part unknown, and is to be gathered only from a careful examination of all the phenomena which seem due to such activity. Here perhaps there stretches before the science of the next generation the unexplored continent which, when explored, may teach us how to wield the powers which heal and save and give life.[1]

4. In the fourth place, nobody can help being struck at once with the decisive power exercised by "faith" as a precondition of Spiritual Healing, and with the variety of the objects which Faith embraces. The most sublime and the most grotesque objects are offered to Faith and accepted by it. It would almost seem, when we look at the facts dealt with by the comparative science of religion, as if it mattered little what we believed in, so long as we did believe whole-heartedly in something. But a little reflection should show that we do not and cannot believe whole-heartedly in anything, cannot have, that is, the faith effective for our purpose, unless we are first sure somehow that the object is worthy of our faith. But worth, or value, is given as a judgment of the transcendental Subject, and not merely of the self-conscious Ego or Person. In

---

[1] It may be instructive to compare with this the statement of an Indian healer given in Appendix D. The attempts of the present writer to secure confirmation of the genuineness of the cures there related have been only partially successful, and therefore the facts there given will have an illustrative value only.

other words, it is a judgment of Reality and not of Appearance, still less of separate interest to the self-conscious Ego. Hence, in general, the object of Faith is the transcendental order, a Power conceived as not merely greater than ourselves, but greater because higher. That is to say, Faith, if not always formally a religious act, is at all events at its highest intensity when it is cast in the religious mould and fed by religious fervour.

This consideration should serve to rescue Faith from the degradation it has suffered in being equated in the popular mind with belief. For even this very belief is vitiated, not merely by being limited to our intellectual power, but still more by being limited to our empirical self as its furthest bound. And it is this last limitation which sets up an effectual barrier against the forces of Spiritual Healing. For all that we have hitherto been discussing points to the invasion of our ordinary sense-consciousness by a power (or powers) which refuses to conform to its rules of experience. A wound according to them should take a month to heal; under Spiritual Healing it takes an hour. A case of *paralysis agitans* is declared incurable, yet it gets itself cured. A cancer disappears and so nullifies the diagnosis. In all these cases, as we have seen reason to believe, a force of a different order from any catalogued in the *Pharmacopeia* intervenes, and the subjective condition for its effectual operation is called Faith.

What then is the nature of this higher Power? We might answer the question by saying that it is the one, omnipresent and unknown Power called

God, who stands over against the world of ordinary consciousness, and seizes the opportunity to intervene and use His power miraculously either when He sees fit arbitrarily, or when the abrogation of self-consciousness permits it. This view, however, is generally, and it would seem rightly regarded now as obsolete. Another and a better answer is that man is a denizen of two worlds at once, and that the two find their meeting-ground in him. He possesses faculties, as the previous pages have sufficiently shown, which transcend the sense-consciousness. This justifies the assertion that he is a transcendental Subject to whom is open both in form and content a cognition superior to that of the sense-consciousness, and not only a cognition, but a power of causation which acts from the higher on to the lower plane of consciousness. That is, the transcendental Subject is also the organizing principle in us, and it distinguishes from itself the empirical Ego which is conscious of pain and disease. In T. H. Green's words man is seen to be "a reproduction of itself by the eternal mind as the self of man to which it makes the process of animal life organic, and which is qualified and limited by the nature of those processes." [1]

Thus it can be proved by the facts of Spiritual Healing that "the soul is richer in ideas than the consciousness, and that the threshold dividing soul and consciousness is movable. Thus also may be understood those phenomena of the soul-life, not less mystical than clairvoyance, and for which physiological explanation leaves always an insoluble

[1] *Prolegomena to Ethics.* Book II. chap. i. § 99.

residue—the will to live, genius and conscience." [1]
By this it comes about that as St. Augustine puts
it: "Man himself is a greater miracle than any
miracle performed by man." [2]
Now the pivotal-point for the understanding of
Spiritual Healing is this truth about the existence
of the transcendental Subject functioning through
our organism, and finding itself on one side helped,
on the other hindered by the organism. And the
problem before us is how to retain the help while
we remove the hindrance. The answer seems to be
that the two states must alternate. Sometimes, for
example, medical science must have our attention
and respectful obedience, but at other times its
limits must be widened and its powers transcended
through the extraordinary activity of the transcendental Subject. Or to put the same proposition
in popular language, sometimes we may be healed
by medical science and sometimes by Spiritual
Healing. Nor is it any part of the duty of those
who serve the latter to deny or belittle the beneficent
operation of the former. In fact, nothing but dis-
aster could be the result of denying the normal
validity of the methods of orthodox medicine, as,

[1] Carl du Prel, *Philosophy of Mysticism*, 1889, ii. 162. *Cf.*
F. W. H. Myers, *Human Personality*, 1907, p. 13: "The
'conscious Self' of each of us, as we call it—the empirical, the
supra-liminal Self, as I should prefer to say—does not comprise
the whole of 'the consciousness' or of the faculty within us.
There exists a more comprehensive consciousness, a profounder
faculty, which for the most part remains potential only so far as
regards the life of earth, but from which the consciousness and
the faculty of earth-life are mere selections, and which reasserts
itself in its plenitude after the liberating change of death."
[2] So: "Et miratur alia, cum sit ipse mirator magnum
miraculum." *Sermo cxxvi.* Bened. ed. v. 614.

for example, Mrs. Eddy in her precipitation has done, just as it is equally unfortunate when orthodox medicine itself, as the therapeutic of the self-conscious, ignores or scoffs at the powers which flow from the transcendental Subject.

But what is the link between the transcendental Subject and the empirical Ego? It is a faculty, at once active and passive, by which the dividing line between the two is shifted, so that more of the riches of the former are exposed for the benefit of the latter. When this shifting of the line assumes a relatively permanent character we call it Conversion or Regeneration, but when it seems to have as its object the removal of some evil felt by the empirical Ego, so that when that specific object is accomplished that Ego proceeds much on its ordinary course, we give it some such name as Spiritual Healing, and we in both cases call the capacity of the Ego for this enlargement and enrichment by the name of Faith. And the true character of an act of faith is best seen when it is described as the act by which the Ego of its own free-will and accord passes from the consciousness of phenomena into the larger consciousness of the transcendental Subject with a corresponding access of power.

This description may help us to appraise the value of the affirmations by which the unwary Christian Scientist is apt to be deceived. He is in some danger of supposing that by virtue of affirming often enough with his self-conscious mind— Mrs. Eddy's mortal mind—his essential holiness, goodness and divinity he may induce immortal

Mind. Of course what he is meant to do is to declare *as* immortal Mind—our transcendental Subject—his true character. But this must have been seen first, and assimilated somehow or other before it can be said as a vital word. And this in its turn demands a previously accepted preparatory discipline. A certain flexibility of the self-conscious Ego must have been acquired by practice before sufficient *vis viva* can spontaneously arise from the depths of the real Being to move the rigid boundaries of self-consciousness further back. Hence the place of self-denial and meditation. To use an illustration favoured by Carl du Prel, we have two consciousnesses rising and sinking like weights in a scale, and they exist contemporaneously, though unconsciously, to each other. It is the practice of thought and contemplation which cultivates the necessary flexibility and produces the man who, in refusing to call himself a Spiritual Healer, shows that he best understands the healing process and his own place in it. If "centuries go to the education and nurture of the wonder-child," as Jean Paul has said, "till it grows up to be the wonder-worker of the world," then some in our midst must be either very young souls, or very old—very young if their work rests on youthful plasticity and spontaneousness, very old, if it is the ripe product of long and varied experience.

This flexibility, however, which is a constitutent factor in the healing process, is prepared for beforehand as all change is. And in this connection one very important branch of curative gymnastic may be singled out for special notice. We refer to the disciplining of the five disturbing passions of Fear, Anger, Lust, Envy and Jealousy. Of these Fear is the passion of the greatest extension, exercising the most widely spread devastating influence on the inner life, and acting as the commonest predisposing condition for disease. So common is its action, so insidious and for the most part so unsuspected by its victim, that even a careful observer is tempted sometimes to conclude that at least in civilized society a man who could shake off all fear would at the same time shake off all liability to disease as well. For fear acts as a dark cloud hiding from view the sun of joyous and buoyant Life, which keeps organs and functions alike in their normal condition of smooth working and healthy contentment. The effect of Fear in impeding the action of the vaso-motor system is unfortunately familiar to everybody, and it is enough to upset the whole organism if it is allowed to be at work over a long period. For Spiritual Healing, therefore, it is necessary that a course of self-discipline be strenuously and persistently undertaken for the purpose of keeping out of the Mind all suggestions arising from Fear. And what is true of Fear is true of all five passions.

The reason of this will be obvious so soon as we remember that the process of Spiritual Healing springs from the transcendental Self, and that that is impeded by all accentuation of the independent activity of the empirical Ego. But the most enduring and most pernicious effect of indulgence in any of the five passions in question is this very accentuation, and the way of physical salvation, therefore, lies through the attenuation of their activity, and so far as possible in their banishment, or, better still, their absorption in a higher spiritual emotion.

5. We have already shown why the word "suggestion" is often made to bear a weight under which it breaks down. To say with the Clerical and Medical Committee of 1914 that suggestion covers all the cases of Spiritual Healing brought before it is just to say nothing. "Suggestion" by itself neither does that nor anything else, any more than the floggings in which the more harsh of our judges (and, alas! some of our bishops) are so childishly credulous have in themselves any improving efficacy. All that is done by suggestion is to ring an alarm-bell. What the man proceeds to do when he is so alarmed depends entirely on what he is, and that again depends on the sort of life he has been living, and especially on the strength of the barriers he has erected physically and psychically between his empirical Ego and himself as a transcendental Subject. In just the same way we print certain words such as Telepathy, Electricity, Functional, Mechanical, and then pin them as labels on certain groups of perceptions without letting ourselves suppose that they tell us anything about the nature of the causes which give us the perceptions. So "suggestion" sets going the machinery, but it does not tell us what the machine is going to turn out, or how it will do it. It is apt, however, to be mistaken by the thoughtless as something more than a name used for convenience of practical life and to be treated as a synthetic judgment by which it is thought some addition is made to our stock of

knowledge about Reality. And this is how it seems to have been used by the Committee. They have confounded the logical distinction between an occasion and a cause.

This question of the relation of suggestion to the healing Life-power in the patient is so important for a right understanding of the problem of Spiritual Healing, that we may be allowed to illustrate it by a reference to its place in a theory of knowledge. We are immediately conscious of our own existence alone, and "all our information as to an external world depends upon ideas which are only changing conditions of ourselves," and the conviction is generally held that our ideas arise from action and reaction with a world independent of ourselves. Now, as Lotze, says, "Wherever action and reaction take place, the nature of the one element is never transferred, identical and unchanged, to the other; but that first element is but as an occasion which causes the second to realize one single definite state out of the many possible for it—that state, namely, which according to the general laws of the nature of that second element is the fitting response to that kind and magnitude of stimulus which it has received." [1]

Thus we may suppose the suggestion to be made to a neurasthenic patient that no cause for fear exists for him. This is the stimulus coming from the object to the subject. But it is not to be thought that something passes from the former to the latter, any more than this happens when two billiard balls cannon. Rather it is that a change

[1] *Microcosmus*, ii. 348.

arising in A becomes the cause by reason of which the relation already existing between A and B is changed by B evolving out of its own nature its new state. A here is the suggestor, B the patient, and the change in the patient depends as much on what he himself already is as on the nature of the suggestion.

6. Next, and we should wish to leave this as the emphatic word on an all-too scanty treatment of a great subject, Spiritual Healing should be defined as but a name for Prayer under one of its aspects, and that by no means the least worthy. Perhaps no word, unless it be God or *I*, is used more thoughtlessly or dogmatically than this word *Prayer*. For it is commonly identified with petition for something the petitioner wants, and all wider use of the term is left out of account. Yet in this wider sense not only is petitioning to be called prayer, but so are praise and thanksgiving. And the statement that the prayer of petition befits those living in faith and hope and so on their way to intuitive vision, while praise and thanksgiving befit those who already see God may be allowed to stand so long as it is understood that the distinction is not between "this side" and "that side," but between two differing conditions of the soul here. Further, meditation and contemplation are important branches of prayer in this wider sense. The former is the dwelling of the mind for practical purposes on some aspect of truth so that it may make the truth at home and familiar, and so dispose itself to assimilate it. The latter is a state or act of the mind by which in different degrees it passes

through every stage from discourse of reason, through immediate vision, up to that ecstasy by which the conscious self gives place to the transcendental Subject, and attains in some sense that union with the Whole which is often called the Mystic Marriage of the Soul.

But for our present purpose it is enough to emphasize one constant factor of every degree of Prayer, whether higher or lower, and that is Desire. This appears to be an integral part of all live Prayer, and to it more than to any other element must be ascribed the faculty by which the soul passes into the condition to which Spiritual Healing is possible. "Hoc licet orare quod licet desiderare" is a word of St. Thomas's (after Augustine) which not only determines the objects for which Prayer may be properly made, but also lets us into the secret of what Prayer essentially is. It is desire, and desire is always the stretching-out of the soul after something it has not got, but feels to be necessary to its satisfaction. And since every yearning of a living thing seems to be the subjective condition necessary for its evolution—that is, for its passing by epigenesis or what not to a higher, that is, a more complex state of existence, so the desire of the soul, which is the pulsing heart of all Prayer, fits that soul for growth into a more complex organic condition.[1]

It may be not unnaturally objected to this pre-

[1] Cessas in vota precesque
Tros ait, Ænea, cessas?   Neque enim ante dehiscent
Adtonitæ magna ora domus.
                              Vergil, Æneid, vi. 52.

sentation of the matter that it reduces prayer to a mechanical exercise of our psychical machinery, and confines it within the area of our own being, and thus excludes the independent action of God as of a Power external to the soul. In reply to this it must be said that its fallacy lies in the spatialization of our concepts about God and the soul. "External" may be the best word at our service to set out the desired view, and yet it may be more misleading than useful. God is not external either to the empirical Ego or to the transcendental Subject. He is to be regarded as the circle with centre everywhere and circumference nowhere, towards which the small circle of the personal Ego and the larger circle of the individuated Subject tend to approach, in order that they may finally identify themselves with it, or, better still, as the common centre of both and of everything else. The language is still mathematical and, therefore, spatial, but at all events it sounds less misleading than the word "external." And the true answer, therefore, to the objection just stated is that our Ego is not a closed self with God outside, but is the organism of our Higher Self or transcendental Subject, which in its turn is a finite centre, and, because it exists at all, a necessary centre of the infinite Being.

7. In Spiritual Healing it is at bottom indifferent whether we distinguish or not medical, mesmeric, mental, spiritualistic or religious modes of healing one from the other, if we understand that all alike derive their efficacy from the one Life which underlies all forms of existence without losing anything of its unity or its peculiar creative power. Mesmerism or animal magnetism are both obnoxious terms,

the former having the fatal defect of being derived from personal peculiarities, while the second assumes improperly that magnetism and animal magnetism are related as inorganic and organic chemistry. It is probable that the force, whatever its nature (and of its existence and limited effectiveness there can be no reasonable doubt), is what is denoted in Hindoo terminology by Prâna, or the cosmic breath. In any case it is the divine Life which seems in gifted hands to be stirred up by physical contact in some form or other, and may be regarded as the most rudimentary form of Spiritual Healing. It may not be impertinent to suggest that medical men might do worse, if they do not themselves practise this particular form of healing, than to employ those who have it, in precisely the same way that they employ anæsthetists, nurses or masseurs. This would at once enlarge the restricted field of medical practice and protect the public from pretenders, and would probably be welcomed by many who at present use their gift in a more or less furtive and disconnected way.

As to mental healing, the term is a complete misnomer if it is intended to suggest that Mind, as thought apart from feeling and will, or even as embracing the whole self-conscious Ego, is competent to perform Spiritual Healing at all. On the contrary, all Spiritual Healing proper depends on the success with which the barriers of that Ego are crossed. Whether the resulting condition is one of ecstasy, hypnosis, or catalepsy generally makes no essential difference provided that it be the condition for the emergent activity of the Higher Self. "Immortal Mind" is the Thinker who transcends our

conscious thinking, and He (or It) is the healer of
our souls and bodies. If this be understood there
is no objection to our using the name mental healing. But on the whole it is more open to miscon-
ception than the term we have used throughout,
viz. *Spiritual Healing*.

With regard to the remaining term "spiritualistic
healing" we need not be detained long. Properly
speaking there is no such thing, for any healing
that may be done through the agency of excarnate
spirits is not done by them at all. Just as the
medical man who makes "suggestions" is but, as
it were, pointing to the direction in which the healing benefit may be sought and found, so any direction given by "spirits" through a medium or to a
patient in a mediumistic condition is but the external
stimulus whose whole potency is exhausted when
it has awakened the sleeping Divinity into curative
action. The animal organism into which our true
Self is partially plunged has its rights even against
its own Subject, and one of those rights is its freedom from compulsion from other Subjects. God,
the great Healer, compels none and invades none
when once He has submitted Himself to the forms
He has chosen to be his organs, and, therefore, all
spirits, incarnate or not, have to respect the inner
sanctuary each of the other. Each may "suggest"
to the other, but none can do more than endeavour
to persuade his fellow to let the Divine in him cure
him of his trouble.

Perhaps the faith of the Spiritual Healer could
hardly be put better than it was put by the late
Mr. F. W. H. Myers, with whose words these
conclusions may fitly close.

"Absolute as the old the new faith might perhaps become if psychological therapeutics should win their assured place by the side of physiological; if it should be recognized that here, too, our appeal is made to no chance caprice, or uncertain favour, but to inflexible and eternal Law. Then, perhaps, the most scientific man would be the most confident, and it would be the sign of wisdom to seek self-healing with the directness of a child. Or is it possible that something beyond mere logical conviction may be needed for the profounder cure; that the Self-healing must needs be felt to depend ultimately on something behind and above the Self? It may be that the inmost effort must still be a religious one, and that to change man deeply it needs a touch upon that mainspring deep in man. What then, for such a purpose, must the religion of science mean? It must mean at least the ancient acceptance of the Universe as good, the ancient sense of the individual effort as co-operant with a vaster Power. If science can regain this sense for man she may do with him what she will. For she will have united with the wonder-solving analysis, the wonder-working faith, and with the wisdom of the children of this world the wisdom of the children of light" (*Proceedings of S.P.R.*, vol. ix. p. 209).

Here we might be content to stop, were it not for the frequency with which from many quarters the term "miracle" is used as the only possible explanation of the marvels of Spiritual Healing. Few of those who use the term seem to have given themselves the trouble of examining it, and it seems necessary, therefore, for us to justify our refusal to accept it as a *vera causa*.

R

CHAPTER XII

THE MIRACULOUS

THE last explanation of the cures wrought by Spiritual Healing is that which goes under the name of the "miraculous." The difficulty involved in this explanation is twofold, and consists partly in ascertaining the sense in which the word is used, and partly in accepting the resulting sense when all others have been rejected. It is necessary, therefore, first of all to inquire into the senses in which the word "miraculous" is used.

Hume, as is well known, held that "a miracle is a violation of the laws of nature; and as a firm and unalterable experience has established these laws, the proof against a miracle, from the very nature of the fact, is as entire as any argument from experience can possibly be imagined. . . . No testimony is sufficient to establish a miracle, unless the testimony be of such a kind that its falsehood would be more miraculous than the fact which it endeavours to establish. Or, briefly, it is contrary to experience that a miracle should be true, but not contrary to experience that testimony should be false." [1]

But the question is, what does Hume mean here

---

[1] Hume is probably responsible for the popular view that (to use his words) a miracle is a transgression of a law of nature by a particular volition of the Deity, or by the interposition of some invisible agent. *Cf.* T. H. Green, *Works*, ed. Nettleship, 1908, i. 276.

by experience? If he means all possible experience, then we have not had it. If he means the general experience of mankind, then all he urges is that to that experience miracles are rare, but not that they are impossible. If, again, he means any given man's experience, then the ground is too narrow for a denial of what other men may have experienced or might experience.

Though Hume will always occupy a high place in the history of philosophy, and his thought be of permanent value for its antiseptic properties, yet his rationalistic or deistic view of the world, in being discredited, has also made his proofs against miracles obsolete as well. But the polemic has been taken up by different, but not wholly dissimilar, philosophies. One of these is Pantheism, especially in the form of Spiritual Monism, of which Spinoza may be regarded as the father in modern philosophy. According to him, all the processes of the universe are manifestations of its Spiritual Life, *natura naturata* being the external form in which *natura naturans* declares itself. Hence, as "nothing happens in nature which is in contradiction with its universal laws," it is clear that a miracle, defined as an event which does contradict these laws, is impossible. Such miracles do not happen.

But what does Spinoza mean by Nature? Does he mean the world as distinct from God, and as a closed whole which shuts out any direct action of God? In this sense miracles certainly become impossible, but it is not Spinoza's sense. Or does he mean that Nature is the comprehensive sum-total of all existence, material and spiritual, embracing

all force, physical and vital, human and divine?
This, which is in accord with his philosophy as a
whole, does not exclude miracles necessarily, unless
we assume that God is subject through the whole
extent of His activity to the mechanical necessity
we detect in Nature.

This assumption, however, is often made by the
Naturalistic School, especially in its evolutionary
doctrine. According to this doctrine, as taught by
Mr. Herbert Spencer, evolution is a rhythmic movement for ever oscillating between homogeneity and
heterogeneity, differentiation and integration, according to inherent laws mechanically acting, with
an otiose Unknowable as the First Great Cause in
the background. Here, again, there is no room
for miracles.

But the strongest ground for the modern dislike
of miracles lies in the implicit belief, which science
has rooted deep in the modern mind, that Nature's
workings are of a uniform character. Thought has
through centuries produced a cosmos out of chaos,
a finite order out of an infinite disorder; and we
are invited, is the complaint, to undo this work and
open the temple of science to potential ruin by
introducing a factor, the miraculous, which can
have no place in this ordered whole. The answer
to this complaint is twofold.

Firstly, it confuses the category of causality with
the uniformity of Nature, and assumes that when
the latter is violated the former is destroyed, which
is not only absurd, but a contradiction in terms.
For all that the Principle of Causality says is that
every change must have a cause; it does not say

that by itself it knows anything of *this* cause necessarily producing *that* effect. Such an affirmation is a conclusion come to by science applying, among other principles, that of Causality. It does not inhere in that principle, which, so far as it goes, coheres as well with an effect miraculously produced as with one that is the result of the mechanical and uniform working of the forces of Nature.

Secondly, as M. Bergson has taught us, the true correlation is not between order and disorder, but between this kind of order and that kind of order.[1] When we expect one kind of order and find another we call what we find disorder, when really all that it is is an order which disappoints our expectations. Hence, when we expect with the Naturalistic School a world explicable in terms of mechanical processes logically concatenated, and find to our surprise that a troublesome and tricksy spirit called a "Miracle" is also there refusing to be so explained, we call out that this "Miracle" introduces disorder into our fair and well-regulated home, whereas all that it does is to invite us to substitute another kind of order, one where "Miracle" finds a niche, in place of the present order, in which "Miracle" has no place. This, of course, says nothing so far as to the substantial character of "Miracle," whether it has, indeed, any substance at all, or whether it is an airy nothing, a mere hallucination. The question of fact still remains untouched.

[1] The two kinds of "order" (each of which may be regarded as a "disorder" to the other) with which M. Bergson is concerned are the physical or geometrical and the vital or willed. The former gives the repetition of similars and the latter redintegration. *Creative Evolution*, p. 236 ff.

Before we approach any question of fact, however, we have still to determine the sense which the champions of miracles attach to that word. For all that has been said so far is of a negative character alone, in that it has suggested that the denial of miracles is not justified except on grounds which assume what ought to be proved. That is, Naturalism assumes that the Universe is a closed universe, or that it is mechanical only, or that our experience is exhaustive in the sense that we can say of any new thing that it is impossible. All which are matters which have to be proved—if they are, indeed, capable of proof.

What, now, do people mean when they maintain not only that miracles have happened, but that they do still happen, or at least may happen? We may for our purpose, and especially after the examples of Spiritual Healing given in the preceding chapters, neglect the once famous superstition which held that miracles happened within Biblical times, but have never happened before or since. Such a destruction of the continuity of the world was never necessary, and would be to-day wanton. The Lord's arm has never been shortened. If He at any time saw fit to work "miracles," reason would rather bid us expect that He would do so again, given the need and the fitness, and not that He would not. But the question is one of fact and of evidence, not of principle.

It will not be improper, perhaps, to take Roman Catholics as the typical champions of the miraculous, seeing that their testimony to it has been the most consistent and is still the most uncompromising. They are content to follow St. Thomas Aquinas for the philosophy of "miracles." And hence we may for the moment follow him. He first replies to the question whether God can do anything beyond the order imposed on things by distinguishing between the order of things as dependent on the First Cause and as dependent on any secondary cause. God cannot, he says, go beyond the former, for in so doing He would be contradicting either His foreknowledge, or His will, or His goodness. But He can go beyond the second order, for it is subject to Him, not He to it, and it is subject "not by necessity of nature, but by the fiat of His will." [1] The distinction, however, does not seem to possess much efficacy, for the order of things being once established, we must needs think of it as not to be set aside without casting a slur on either the Divine wisdom, or power, or goodness. God, who *simpliciter* could do what He chose, cannot *ex suppositione*, on the supposition that He has lent to the course of things something of His own reality, something, therefore, which in its very being partakes of His wisdom, power and goodness. In this sense, then, we may say that God can go "præter ordinem rebus inditum," but not "contra ordinem rebus inditum." That is to say, He is to be thought of as respecting the *ordo* He Himself has put here, and therefore as doing nothing to violate it, but He is not to be thought of as exhausting His powers by that *ordo*,

---

[1] *Summa*, 1. cv. 6 : talis ordo ei subjicitur, quasi ab eo procedens, non per necessitatem naturæ, sed per arbitrium voluntatis.

but as still reserving the right to go beyond it, by carrying it still further, or by adding to it further powers, and so taking it towards perfection. Thus we might think of man's "freedom" as not a violation of Nature's necessity, but as that towards which Nature was unconsciously pressing on; just as we regard regeneration as transcending while using and so confirming the principle of generation.

When St. Thomas comes to ask whether everything that God does beyond the natural order of thing is a miracle, he replies [1] that the term miracle comes from admiration—"miraculum ab admiratione"—and that this admiration or wonder takes place when the effects are plain and the cause is hidden. But the cause may be hidden from some and be known to others; hence, *e. g.* an eclipse may be a *miraculum* to the rustic and not to the astronomer. The word *miraculum*, therefore, should be restricted to what is fully admirable, whose cause is hidden from all. Such a cause is God alone. Hence "those things which come to pass from God beyond causes known to us are called miracles." [2] In this view St. Thomas agrees formally with Spinoza, whose "unknown" law was to the effect that the term "miracle" was to be applied to an event which we are unable to explain

---

[1] *Summa*, i, cv. 7.

[2] Illa quæ a Deo fiunt præter causas nobis notas miracula dicuntur. With this agrees Augustine : "Portentum fit, non contra naturam sed contra quam est nota natura." *De Civ. Dei,* xxi. 8, § 2. *Cf.* "The word 'miracle' is used here in its etymological sense to denote something marvellous and opposed to common experience, that at first sight cannot be accounted for by the agency of natural causes." *Brit. Med. Journal,* June 18, 1910, p. 1483.

by other events familiar to our experience. He differs from Spinoza in the freedom He assigns to God to bring out of His treasures new things.[1]

St. Thomas then proceeds to maintain that some miracles are greater than others, not in respect of the power performing them, but in respect of their effects. He makes a threefold classification : (a) quoad substantiam facti, (b) quoad id in quo fit, and (c) quoad ad modum. The *first* class includes all wonders which are beyond the powers of Nature altogether, as when the sun goes backward, or when the human body is glorified. The *second* class includes wonders of a lower degree, wonders, that is, which Nature might work, but not in the subjects where they occur, as the raising of the dead, the giving sight to the blind; for Nature can be the cause of life, but not to a dead man, and can give sight, but not to a blind man. The *third* class includes wonders of a still lower degree, in which things are done within the compass of Nature's powers, but in a way surpassing Nature's way. Cures that are instantaneous in cases where Nature usually requires a considerable space of time come under this head.[2]

Further, a miracle may be wrought (a) through God's own immediate action, or (b) mediately. Under (b) would come angels, men and inanimate things. And again, a miracle is always a sign.[3]

---

[1] *Cf.* Cum naturæ ordo sit a Deo rebus inditus, si quid præter nunc ordinem faciat non est contra naturam, *Summa*, I, cv. 6, ad 1.

[2] *Summa*, I, cv. 8.

[3] τέρατα *wonders*, σημεῖα *signs*, δυνάμεις *powers*, are associated in the New Testament.

Hence the miracle is addressed to the reason, including the moral judgment; it is a sign of the imminence of the higher or super-sensual world. Therefore it is differentiated by its purpose from trickery, magic, and all mere displays of skill or of "occult" power. "The *wonder* shows the miracle as a deviation from the ordinary course of nature, the *sign* gives the purpose of the deviation."

From this it is now clear that those who affirm miracles do so by connecting them at once with Nature and with God. With Nature, because without her order nothing would be held to be wonderful, since all would be equally surprising. With God, because without His free action there is no reason why Nature should not be thought of as a tedious "repetition of similars," instead of being a continuous series of acts of creation, where some acts are more wonderful than others. But in this relation of the miracle to Nature and of the miracle to God, they are more concerned with the latter than with the former. On the other hand, scientists and philosophers are more concerned with the former relation. They are jealous for the unity and order of the world, and are less interested in it as the reflection of God, while men of religion feel it to be their first care to preserve the autonomy of God, and so to ensure the possibility of a personal relation between the soul and God. It may be that the two knights see the shield from two different sides, and so describe it differently, and that both sides may be at once true and important.

If, then, the thinker suspects the word miracle as connoting an *arbitrary* exercise of God's power, he can appeal to the popular use of the word to justify his suspicion. And, indeed, this would seem to be what people ordinarily mean by a miracle. But this is not the meaning which the thoughtful man of religion puts on it. He means by a "miracle" some happening in the sensible world in which God is the prime actor, whether He work through the orderly course of things or in some exceptional manner, in which we cannot trace the sensible effects to their first cause. It is true that theologians are careful to point out that they do not call God's ordinary workings miracles, even though they are beyond the powers of Nature, such as the creation of souls, the Eucharistic miracle, and the graces which flow from the Sacraments. It is not easy to see, however, why they should abstain from extending the sweep of the miraculous thus far. The wonders of the world, whether of nature or of grace, are wonders wrought by God, and there is nothing but our ignorance or stolidness which makes the extraordinary more wonderful than the ordinary. That the sun rises every morning is in reality a much more wonderful, if less startling, thing than if he sometimes did and sometimes did not. That a skilful physician can diagnose a complicated malady accurately and cure in twelve months what has been coming on for years is, when calmly considered, as marvellous as when a man like de Rudder is cured instantaneously. Nothing is gained by restricting the marvellous to the exceptional, and the implication that the exceptional is the *arbitrary*, that is, the uncaused, is responsible for the hostility of all sound thinkers to a doctrine which must seem to them to cut at the very tap-root of the Tree of Truth. As Mr. McTaggart says: "If we conceive change without causation we reduce the universe to chaos—which is certainly not compatible with the Absolute Idea."[1]

The question, then, as to the nature of the power which manifests itself in Spiritual Healing is not to be disposed of merely by calling it miraculous. G. H. Lewes once wrote, for example, that "when any man says that phenomena are produced by *no* known physical laws, he declares that he knows the laws by which they are produced."[2] That is to say, if the laws of the universe are divisible into *a* (the known) and *not-a* (the unknown), then if a man says that Spiritual Healing is inexplicable by *a* he declares that he knows *not-a*, that is, he knows the unknown. Which is absurd, and is contradicted, too, by the Roman Catholic apologist. Such a man asserts that in "miracles" such as those of Lourdes "the connection between cause and effect is cancelled to such an extent that the same water, used as a bath or a lotion, now fills up a pair of hollow lungs, now heals up caries or cures an abdominal inflammation."[3]   Indeed, Catholic

---

[1] *Studies in Hegelian Cosmology*, 1901, p. 29.

[2] Report of Dialectical Society's Committee on *Spiritualism*, 1873, p. 230.

[3] Jörgensen, *Lourdes*, p. 183. Jörgensen also says : "The miraculous is closely related to dogma. Christian doctrines, for instance, about the Trinity, about the Virgin Birth of Jesus, His Resurrection, His Ascension, are rejected by many because they are unthinkable. This is true, they *are* unthinkable. We can accept these sentences as correct, *i.e.* corresponding to actual facts, but we cannot connect them with any concrete idea in our minds."

piety seems to exult in the fact that its miracles defy all explanation, and it certainly is scornful of any suggestion that they may some day be seen to be subject to Law, Law which at present remains unknown.

At the opposite pole we find a flat denial that "miracles" in any tolerable sense of that word are possible at all. "Let us ask what is involved in the conception of a cause not acting uniformly; we shall see that it is the same as if we denied the existence of causal connections altogether."[1] But it is just the conception of a Cause not acting uniformly which is the conception maintained by those who appeal to Miracles. And it is this conception of "a sudden and unexpected jerk, as it were, of the Almighty hand that controls the machinery of the universe "[2] which is the current and widespread superstition which alone we are concerned to combat. Mr. Rawlinson goes on to say on the page from which we have just quoted that "the best definition of a miracle is that it is something which, when we are confronted by it, compels us to say, ' This is the Lord's doing, and it is marvellous in our eyes.' " Unfortunately this is more of a description than a definition, and we get a clearer account of the popular view in Mr. Temple's Essay in the same volume,[3] in which he says, "A hundred and fifty years ago it was generally supposed that God had made the world and then left it to behave according to laws He had imposed, interfering now and then by way of

---

[1] Joseph, *Introduction to Logic*, p. 374.
[2] *Foundations*, p. 167.   [3] p. 243.

miracle; God acted, in short, here and there, now and then."

It would seem, therefore, that from the side of Christian Apologetic we have to meet a doctrine of miracles which is no longer vital, but merely a survival from the obsolete Deism of the Age of Enlightenment. Just as it is impossible to talk of miracles when there is no sense of continuity,[1] so it is equally impossible to talk of miracles as "sudden interruptions of the established order by occasional interferences of divine power," or as embodying the "idea of complete fortuitousness and arbitrariness," in an age which has drunk deep of the doctrine of the coherence and unity of the universe.

It is this coherence and unity which the scientific and philosophic worlds hold themselves bound in honour to maintain against the arbitrariness which seems engrained in popular religious thought. Indeed, we may say that here the philosopher is more spiritual in his teaching than the preacher, as when Mr. Bosanquet says, "Where there is (or appears to be) discontinuity . . . there inevitably is (or appears to be) *pro tanto* a gap in the embodiment of spiritual purpose and significance. A purpose is not realized, it is not a reality as penetrating and vivifying a mass of content, if it is not affirmed continuously and traceably in a coherent structure. No purpose or significance can be realized through

[1] "It is only to the modern conception of Nature that a miracle could seem really miraculous, for this conception recognizes no impulse of which the result does not follow necessarily and according to general laws, from a pre-existing collocation of conditions." Lotze, *Microcosmus*, ii. 478.

miracle." [1] The true spiritual ideal demands mechanical intelligibility; both factors are somehow true at the same time; and mechanical intelligibility ceases to be directly we admit interventions, exceptions and uncaused change.[2]

Again, then, we inquire whether the hostility between the philosophic denial of miracle and the fervid advocacy of miracle by pious feeling is necessary. We think it is not. The former is contending for the *rationality* of God in the world, and the latter for the *freedom* of God in the world. The only miracle which the former banishes is that which destroys coherency. The only mechanism which the latter denies is that which enslaves God as the Lord of Life. And the difficulty which piety puts in the way of philosophy is caused by its separating two things which God has joined together, viz. Spirit and Mechanism. It has regarded the mind, plan, teleology or purpose in the Universe as outside it, as it were, an *extra* brought in to complete it, instead of being a constituent part of its very being, in the same way that man's spirit is a constituent part of what he is as one continuous and indivisible whole.

Mr. Bosanquet protests against "this separation of the whole from the guiding element " which is involved in the vulgar view of matter *plus* miracle,

---

[1] *The Principle of Individuality and Value,* 1912, p. 141.

[2] " Of the two points of view, it is impossible for either to be entirely absent.' Assuming this possibility to be possible, a total failure of mechanical intelligibility would reduce the spiritual to the miraculous, the negation of all spirituality, as a total failure of teleological intelligibility would reduce individuality to incoherence and annihilate mechanism." B. Bosanquet *loc. cit.,* p. 155 f.

"the attitude of common external teleology by which the 'plan' is brought to the material; is not in it or elicited from it."[1]

This notion of soul and body, spirit and matter, mechanism and teleology being forces allied indeed as pairs, but external to one another and at bottom hostile, is responsible for the fog in which the idea of Miracle is involved for both science and theology. The fog, however, lifts so soon as we replace this false dichotomy by the judgment which affirms not God *and* Nature, but God *in* Nature. "Nature as a whole can neither stand still nor cease to correspond to the meaning of the One of which all its active elements are but dependent emanations. In it, therefore, must be accomplished the task of a perpetual preservation, not merely of some order, but of the order contained in the meaning of its first creation."[2] To suppose that any new order introduced, instead of carrying forward the order first of all imposed on Nature, contradicts it and sets it aside is to say that God has by His later action contradicted His former action,[3] which is absurd. But, on the other hand, we cannot regard the order of Nature as static, but rather as displaying a moving equilibrium—moving, that is, along the path prescribed from the first by the Reason or Wisdom inherent in Nature. We say "inherent in Nature" in order to exclude the con-

---

[1] *The Principle of Individuality and Value*, 1912, p. 205.

[2] Lotze, *Microcosmus*, i. 449.

[3] Ea vero quæ contradictionem implicant, sub divina omnipotentia non continentur, quia non possunt habere possibilium rationem. St. Thomas Aq., *Summa*, Ia, xxv. 3. St. Thomas adds that that which involves a contradiction cannot be true because no intellect can think it.

cept of Nature being a machine set going, but requiring from time to time correction by the hand of intelligence brought to bear from outside on the machine in order to save it from its own blind blunders. It is this concept of intelligence and mechanism being two independent forces which is responsible for the vulgar idea of miracle as an arbitrary interference with the order of Nature. But if we come to see that the mechanism is itself intelligent, or, if the phrase be preferred, is the expression of an indwelling intelligence, we get rid, indeed, of the arbitrariness of miracle, but not of the Divine freedom working through it. And it is this latter which alone religion is concerned with, just as it is the former which alone philosophy is bound to combat.

No philosopher is better fitted to help us to reconcile these two distinct though complementary views than Lotze, and that not merely because he was by temperament and conviction a mediator.[1] He combined in himself a singular power of broad and comprehensive as well as original constructive thought, together with a religious warmth of feeling; and the two, the thought and the feeling, instead of neutralizing, only enriched one another. Lotze does not refuse to allow the miracle in some sense, but he is careful to mark out that sense. He would not use the term for what was unusual but in its commencement calculable, for this would

[1] "Lotze's problem is to reconcile oppositions, or to mediate between contrary opinions. It is a synthetic reconstruction of philosophy which will take account of all departments of knowledge." E. P. Robins, *Some Problems of Lotze's Theory of Knowledge* in "*Cornell Studies in Philosophy*," 1900, p. 8. The same was true of Kant.

S

narrow too much the signification of the word. On the other hand, he is equally averse to a view of miracle which would regard it as a complete setting aside of the laws of Nature. For if this took place not only would the single event called the miracle be made possible, but it would take place at the expense of the order of the rest of the world, "whose orderly and regular continued existence we presupposed as the foil for the lustre of the single miracle." But if we are to be allowed to admit at all any partial annulling of a law of Nature, this can only be when we have first established the interdependence of the inner and the outer sides of Nature. "The miracle-working power, whatever it may be, does not directly turn against the law to set aside its authority, but by altering the inner states of things, in virtue of its internal connection with them, it indirectly modifies the usual result of the law, whose validity it leaves intact and permanently turns to account. The complete and unbending circle of mechanical necessity is not, and must not be, immediately accessible to the miracle-working command; but the inner nature of that which is subject to its laws is determined not by it, but only by the meaning of the universe." [1]

We are to regard, then, as the sole legitimate sense of the term "miracle" that which means by it a sensible event of a striking character which proceeds from the indwelling Life and is a moment— "a phase which remains an element"—in that Life as a progressive and consistent movement towards an end which is itself inherent in the movement. This definition may sound cumbrous, but a little

[1] *Microcosmus,* i. 451.

consideration will show that each clause of the definition is necessary. For (a) the miracle must be at least a sensible event; it is in "ultimates," as Swedenborg would say. The unseen ground of the order or purpose in Nature is not a miracle, it is a mystery, though the mystery might at any moment become a miracle by coming out of its lair. And (b) it is of a striking character, for otherwise we should be under the necessity of obliterating the distinction between what is to us ordinary and what is to us extraordinary by regarding all events alike as miraculous on account of their wonderfulness. And so we should get rid of the miracle as such. Again (c) the miracle proceeds from the indwelling Life, for otherwise we should be once more driven to the concept impossible to philosophy of a Universe governed by intermittent jerks applied from outside. And (d) the changes introduced from within in the order of Nature must spring (for everybody who regards the world as rational) from an end or value in the order itself. For otherwise, the end defined as a *terminus ad quem* in arriving gives satiety as the end of conation in place of the satisfaction which accompanies and measures the value of the whole conative process. In other words, the "end" of a miracle is in the miracle itself, and the whole value of the miracle would be destroyed if the reason for its being performed lay wholly outside of it. When de Rudder's broken leg was miraculously healed [1] this was not to prove the truth of Roman Catholic doctrine or the reality of Bernadette's visions, but merely because a universe with a broken leg

[1] p. 108

in it is less valuable or desirable than one without it.

We seem now to be in a position to understand why the Roman Catholic advocates so strenuously the concept of miracle as a supernatural act of God. What he wants to effect by this contention is acceptance for his belief in God's freedom and in His personal activity. And he thinks that anybody who refers the "miracle" to an unknown natural cause is thereby pledged to the exclusion of God by assigning the whole activity displayed in the "miracle" to the forces of the Nature which he has begun by setting over against God.[1] But, as we have seen already, to separate God and Nature is a philosophical blunder. See God *in* Nature, and then you have at once a view of Reality which gives their due both to God's creative freedom and Nature's mechanical intelligibility.

Yet we ought to be grateful to men like Mgr. Benson,[2] M. Jörgensen, Docteur Boissarie and

[1] Thus Georges Bertrin makes his theologian, when instructing the doctor, say that instantaneousness in the restoration of organic tissues will never possibly be a natural fact, whatever may happen or whatever discovery may be made, because it is contrary not only to the laws of the organism but to its very constitution, to its nature, and its essence. Passing by the fallacy involved here in identifying the laws of Nature in general with those known to us in particular, a fallacy which vitiates the whole of M. Bertrin's plea for "miracle" as a supernatural intruder into Nature, we need only say that his further assertion that no natural cause known or unknown is sufficient to account for the marvellous facts seen at Lourdes, introduces in a still more objectionable form the assumption that we know the unknown "natural causes" well enough to assert what they cannot do. But this is ridiculous. *Histoire Critique des Événements de Lourdes,* 1912, pp. 226, 229.

[2] In a very fervid lecture delivered at Caxton Hall on June 22 last, Mgr Benson ridiculed the idea that suggestion could

Georges Bertrin for the very one-sidedness of their contention that "miracle" means that God is at

do what was done at Lourdes, and inquired what difference there was between suggestion in general and religious suggestion except the religion—an epigram which is obviously misleading. For it may mean that the implicit faith of the pilgrim acts as a very subtle and powerful auto-suggestion, which is what "religious suggestion" alone can mean, and what the lecturer did not mean by it. Or it may mean, and this is what Mgr. Benson was concerned to show, the objective working of a Power recognized by religion, but this is not properly included under suggestion at all. He also related several cases of cures, including the case of a woman who had great wounds in her back in 1907, and was cured, utterly and permanently, in the space of a day or two. He saw her in 1908, and an American lady with whom he was travelling examined her, and was able to testify that there had been no return of the malady. He also described the case of a little girl two-and-a-half years of age, blind from her birth. This child was held in the arms of Mme. Carrel, wife of Dr. Carrel, of the Rockefeller Institute, New York, who himself received the Nobel Prize in 1912. Mme. Carrel was a qualified medical woman, and not at all the kind of person to be deceived or imposed on by herself or by others. As the Blessed Sacrament approached in procession she noticed that the child was moving her head, her eyes opened, and she made several attempts to clutch the gold bracelet which Mme. Carrel took from her arm to see if it would attract the child's attention. That, however, was not a complete miracle, and was not regarded as satisfactory by the bureau at Lourdes, where they were very critical and exacting as to evidence.

He had asked Dr. Carrel his opinion of these things, and he had replied that he had come to two absolutely certain conclusions and one uncertain one. The first of his certain conclusions was that no scientific explanations yet framed could account for the phenomena at Lourdes. Mgr. Benson asked Dr. Carrel, "What about suggestion?" He laughed and replied, "All those people who talk about suggestion do not know what they are talking of." The second conclusion was that the cures depended upon the intensity of prayer—that when the wave of prayer rose high then the cures were frequent, and that when it sank low the cures did not take place. Of these two conclusions Dr. Carrel said he was as certain as he was of any scientific fact in the world. What he was not certain of was whether or not vitality was imparted to the afflicted by those who sympathized with them in the multitude of the whole people present. If it were so, said Mgr.

work, for, after all, this assertion of theirs is far nearer the truth of things than the denial of God's activity implicit in Hume's famous sentence, and, what is more, it does greater justice than most other explanations to the full meaning of the "miracle" as at once a portent, a sign and a power. As a portent it is a wonder; as a sign it points to the spiritual order; and as a power it maintains that God working in Nature is our help and strength. All three factors are necessary to the full force of the term "miracle."[1] It would be well if "miracle" in the thoroughly defensible sense of Lotze could be replaced by some term which would not connote the arbitrariness with which "miracle" is inextricably associated in ordinary language; but as there is little prospect of such a term being found, or of its winning general acceptance if found, we must perforce continue to use the term, while explaining carefully the sense we put on it.

Hence we may conclude that we may legitimately attribute the cures wrought at Lourdes and elsewhere to miraculous agency, if by that phrase we intend the direct intelligent action of God as the indwelling Power in Nature which (while continuously carrying Nature onward by Itself becoming outward) from time to time makes its normal working remarkable by some feature which is not so much new in itself as new to our usually holden eyes.

Benson, it would not seem contrary to Christian teaching. This last suggestion of Dr. Carrel's, while it points the way to a rational view of the miraculous, seems at the same time to cut away the root of the popular idea of "miracle" as uncaused. The lecture was reported in *The Times* for June 23, 1914.

[1] The three terms, τέρατα *wonders*, σημεῖα *signs*, and δυνάμεις *powers*, are combined in Acts ii. 22 and 2 Thes. ii. 9.

CHAPTER XIII

Spiritual Healing among Primitive Peoples.—It may be convenient to summarize our discussion. We began with a short description of the salient features of medical practice in those stages of civilization (or of the absence of it) which we agree in calling "primitive." In them the power of the medicine-men, the use of incantations, the belief in animism, the practice of magical rites are characteristic. And they all rest on the belief, almost spontaneous, in animism, a belief which for some time has been discredited in modern thought, but yet seems almost a hardy annual by its stubborn resistance to all attempts to extirpate it. Thus Prof. William McDougall's *Body and Mind,* and the Gifford Lectures of Hans Driesch on the *Science and Philosophy of the Organism,* and his little work on the *Problem of Individuality* may be taken as examples of the persistent truth wrapped up in animism. "Naturam expellas furcâ tamen usque recurret." It is true that Dr. Driesch does not speak of animism but of vitalism, nor of "soul" but of "entelechy," but all the same he ranges himself on the side of those who maintain that the wholeness of the individual organism is assured or restored by a non-mechanical process. And it is

263

possible to maintain that the magic of primitive peoples did whatever it did in the way of healing by somehow setting going the vital or non-mechanical processes by which Spiritual Healing is effected.

The main reason, therefore, for insisting on the relevancy of the beliefs and practices of primitive peoples to our subject is that it is a mistake to treat them as mere childish beliefs of the race which we have long outgrown. However great their formal error, they seem to have been substantially right. That is to say, they were dependent on errors of observation, on hasty generalizations, on the Fear which dogs the footsteps of all animal and savage life, but in spite of the imperfect forms to which these evils gave rise, the substantial truth underlying them still holds good, viz. that Life fills all forms and uses all forms, and hence that Spiritual Healing consists in inducing somehow that Life to assert its beneficent activities.

The Greek World.—When we pass to the Greek world we are not changing with our sky our outlook. In the famous cult of Asklepios we find still prevailing the same kind of beliefs and practices as met us among primitive peoples. It is a great spirit, god or demi-god, who through his priests and his cult performs cures, although here one feature, that of incubation, is emphasized. No doubt, however, exists that the healing practised at Epidauros, Cos, Athens and elsewhere in the name of Asklepios belongs rather to Spiritual Healing than to scientific. Prayer and dreams and the general suggestiveness of the place, religious faith, a strong desire and expectancy formed the subjective factors of the cure. But it would seem that the exclusion of any objectively present spiritual being, such as Asklepios was thought to be, would be a sceptical procedure not warranted when a general survey of Spiritual Healing in all ages and countries is undertaken. It is more rational, and now-a-days more philosophical, to look to some spiritual agent as co-operating with the faith of the patient. Which is but to say that our normal experience of subject and object should be extended to cover the phenomena of Spiritual Healing. Whether we call the stimulating agent Asklepios or the Blessed Virgin would seem to be matter of indifference. God fulfils Himself in many ways.

Early Christianity.—No essential difference is to be traced between the cures due to Spiritual Healing in pagan times and in Christian times, for the chief difference between the two dispensations is of a temporal character, the latter taking up the former, and carrying it onward and upward, as takes place in all processes that go on in Time. Before and after the opening of the Christian era men looked to a Saviour-God to heal them both in soul and body. What Asklepios had done Christ also did, and His followers in their turn took over the functions of the Asklepiadæ. Hence the older criticism of the "miracles" of healing ascribed in the Canon to Christ and His earliest followers, is already discredited and out of date. The rationalism of Reimarus and of the German Illuminationists; the naturalism of the English deists; the "mythical" explanation of Paulus; the thoroughgoing "higher criticism " of Strauss have, no doubt, all done useful service to Truth in their time, but that time is past. We now, without forfeiting our critical rights, are better able to allow for a core of solid reality in the stories of the Spiritual Healing attributed to Jesus Christ. Whether He worked through the use of Prâna, or by the suggestion which a strong and living personality can exert on a weak one, or by the conscious or unconscious application of a Force which, in the strict sense, is and remains "supernatural," or by all these ways is a matter for inquiry and discussion. But we no longer reject *a priori* the Biblical stories of supernormal healing, because our attention has been drawn to the undeniable fact that stories of similar happenings in our own days are well grounded. There are more things in heaven and earth than the most thoroughgoing science or the most advanced philosophy knows.

The Middle Age.—We have given what may be thought a quite undue proportion to the "miracles" of the Saints, but on reflection we hope it will be conceded that good grounds exist for studying the *Acta Sanctorum.* To regard them, as was generally done until recently as a mere quarry for folk-lore, is to be unable to see the wood for the trees. It may be freely granted that the imagination of the mystery-monger has been at work to embellish the narratives; that ecclesiastical piety has sometimes jumped to conclusions congenial to it, or sometimes deliberately made truth subservient to the influence of the Church; that very often the form of the "miracle" is obviously borrowed from Biblical antitypes; and that many stories are inherently improbable. But when all is allowed for on the grounds of credulity, interest or fraud, there does seem to remain a considerable number of stories of Spiritual Healing which we are not justified in treating with contempt. And of such we have tried to give some samples.

But the greatest "miracle" of all remains if criticism succeeds in inducing us to abandon all the healing deeds attributed to mediæval saints. For how are we then to account for the fact that the whole of Christendom cherished without questioning its conviction of the possibility and, from time to time, of the fact of the miraculous? It may be urged that the Catholic Church was too strong a body to be questioned with impunity, but this is to forget that the strength of that Church lay in the implicit beliefs of its members, and they all believed in miracles. Or it may be said that the age was an age of faith and not of criticism, that it was, in fact, the Dark Age *par excellence*. But this can only mean that it is dark to us, for there is ample evidence that intellectual thought and inquiry were abundant enough. Even the crusades such as those of De Montfort and the Inquisition were unable to stamp out free thought in the heretical bodies, such as the Cathari, Paterines, Paulicians, the Albigenses, and those loosely grouped together as Manichæans. Nor can we forget the names of Duns Scotus, Peter Abelard, Roger Bacon, John Wycliffe and many other brave men before Martin Luther, all of whom represent an amount of silent intellectual thought which it would be a mistake to ignore.

No, when all allowance is made, there still remains the logical difficulty of understanding how the belief in "miracles" could maintain itself not only in being, but in lusty and strong health for fifteen hundred years, if it had not been constantly fed by actual facts. Those facts may have been less numerous or less wonderful than the mediæval mind believed, and not at all violations of Nature, but at least they must have been something, unless, indeed, we are to think that men are irrational enough to believe through long centuries of change anything they want to believe. Moreover, they were not always inventions of later date, as the "miracles" of St. Thomas of Canterbury show, but were known, testified to and accepted by men who were no more credulous than modern Christians, or, for the matter of that, modern critics.

That the Saints of whose doings we have given some samples were close followers of Pagan wonder-workers, so far from militating against their *bona fides*, really tells *tantum quantum* in its favour. For one great dialectical advantage which accrues from wiping out the false line of demarcation which long use and convenience have drawn between the three last centuries B.C. and the three first centuries A.D., is that it puts us in a position for judging fairly of both. For the merits of Christianity are lessened rather than enhanced by all depreciation of Paganism, seeing that Paganism supplied the materials out of which the living spirit of Christianity constructed its temple. If we are to accept the records of Spiritual Healing in the Middle Age, we shall hardly do so if we begin by ruling out those of pre-Christian Paganism. For if Spiritual Healing be a fact at all, it must be due to a Force which, being of divine origin, never leaves itself without witness wherever the laws of its working allow it to operate.

In fact, it is not by any means a wild conjecture that such a "magnetic personality" as that of Martin of Tours gained adherents because they were themselves objects of his healing-powers. In London to-day it is easy enough to find a dozen "spiritual healers" whose *modus operandi* is obviously that of modifying in some manner the working of that force which in the East is called Prâna. There is no mystery about this method of healing; it is within the reach of scientific formulation, and it is more than probable that striking personalities, such as St. Ubaldo or St. Martin, possessed a natural aptitude for such healing activity, and that they were believed to be able to heal just because they did, as a matter of fact, heal.

Modern Times.—We take, for convenience' sake, modern history, to begin with the reign of Henry VII.[1] And here we seem face to face with a new factor, that of a more lively spirit of criticism, which has apparently succeeded not only in diminishing the number of cases of Spiritual Healing, but also in damping down the expectation of such healing. It would hardly be contended that modern Protestantism is religious in the same sense that Catholicism on the Continent is religious. Both sides

---

[1] A story is told of two successive professors of modern history, one of whom dated it from the French Revolution, and the other from the Call of Abraham.

would affirm this distinction eagerly; and it would seem to be corroborated—with one remarkable exception, that of Christian Science—by the fact that where the Protestant spirit of inquiry and criticism is active, the phenomena of Spiritual Healing are comparatively few. It is not that they are not found, but that they are not found so often, and when they are found they occur where the religious attitude is similar to that which prevails among Catholic peasantry. In this respect the Peculiar People and the Salvation Army are nearer to Catholic Brittany than they are to Canterbury or Geneva. That is to say, where the faith which receives the gift is *fides quâ creditur*, and not merely *fides cui creditur*, to use a convenient formula, there the healing power is more in evidence. Some exceptional amount of expectant emotion, of desire and self-surrender, seems to be the normal subjective factor required before the healing process can be set going. But this is not always necessary, as the curious case of Gabriel Gargam, healed at Lourdes, shows, unless, indeed, here we are to assume that the faith of his friends acted as surrogate for his.

The Lourdes cures seem to stand by themselves in some respect. It is not their number, for the number seems to be relatively small, nor is it the wonders attaching to the foundation of the shrine, nor the piety of the workers, which for our purpose are pertinent. It is the fact that a small number of the cures appear to be paralleled nowhere else; witness the case of Gargam just referred to, and that of de Rudder, which, though performed at

Oostacker, belongs here. When the medical profession insists that Spiritual Healing is applicable
only to functional disease, and is explicable by
suggestion alone, it may be invited to tell us what
it makes of these two cases. Fraud or exaggeration, or doubtful diagnosis, all seem excluded. Both
were cases of undoubted organic lesion, and one
was sceptical. We seem to be in presence of a
Force which at present defies formulation.

One observation may be not out of place on
the instantaneousness which marks these and other
cures. Father Benson and others stake their whole
plea for the miraculousness of the Lourdes' cures
on this very instantaneousness, which they contrast
with the stately slowness of the ordinary processes
of Nature. To us, however, the argument seems
very precarious. It is similar to the argument from
sudden conversion to the miraculous, and like that
seems based on a want of consideration of all the
facts. St. Paul's writings, for example, make it
clear that his conversion was no wholly unprepared
for event, but the climax of a process. Similarly,
we speak of sudden flashes of inspiration, forgetting
altogether the long brooding thought beforehand
which has made the inspiration possible. The
lightning that shines from the east to the west is
apt to startle us by its suddenness, but we forget
that that suddenness is only the mark of our ignorance. We forget the slowly maturing over-
accumulation of electricity in the clouds which has
made the electric flash necessary. We may say
that a thought suddenly occurs to us, when we
ought to say that after long thinking in a more or

less desultory way, our thoughts come to a head in a thought which we find decisive. A sudden resolution is only sudden because we ignore the underground work of the mind in preparing for it. By analogy, therefore, we seem bound to suspect that the argument from the suddenness of the cures at Lourdes to their miraculousness is invalid; it is in all probability based on ignorance of the healing process, which had been set going some time before, but only there came to its full perfection. This consideration, too, might also account for the comparative fewness of the cures effected. The others had not gone through the necessary preliminary steps by which the goal is reached.

Christian Science.—The last of the modes of healing which history tells of, and in some ways the most remarkable, is that known as Christian Science. And an appreciation of it is all the more pressed on us because of the very unlikelihood that such a world-wide movement should proceed from such a founder. Indeed, so ill fitted was Mrs. Eddy by nature, training and temperament for the fine work of Spiritual Healing, that the merits of her system are but enhanced by the earthen character of the vessel from which they were poured out. Moreover, the sacred canon of Christian Science is composed in such uncouth jargon that it is almost a miracle that it should ever have been regarded as inspired. Every page of it has to be translated into the dialect of the spirit before it can set out truth, and the virtue then lies in the trans-lation, not in the original text. Yet in spite of its birth's invidious bar, Christian Science gets home. Its cures are more numerous than those of Lourdes, equally startling by their contempt for all orthodox formulæ, while the spread of the Church of Christ Scientist has no modern parallel, save that of the Salvation Army. Those who believe that both rest at bottom on superstition, must take a gloomy view of human nature when they see how institutions thus batten on it. On the other hand, those who take a nobler and more hopeful view will see in the triumphs of Christian Science another indication of the power of Life to overcome even the most hardened prejudices and most stubborn vested interests.

Spiritual Healing and the Body.—After setting out the evidence for Spiritual Healing as a historical fact, we passed in this chapter (VI) to ask whether the constitution of human nature allows for any place to such healing, and if so, how we are to conceive its method of working. And here we were faced by an ambiguity in the meaning of the Soul. According to popular terminology this term denotes an intermediary third to Spirit and Body, whereas analysis would seem to show that Soul (or Mind) and Body are two aspects of one and the same mechanism, which mechanism as a whole is at the service of a timeless Self or transcendental Subject. This mechanism, involving as it does life and purpose, seems to possess in itself some degree of self-adjustment, or self-recovery, and these processes may well come under the head of Spiritual Healing, and specifically of mental self-healing, if we desire to be more explicit.

T

This led us to examine the now common term sub-conscious, and to hesitate a doubt as to whether it was not made to cover too much material, whether, for example, it was identical with Mr. Myers's "subliminal Self," or was some lesser or different thing. Mr. Myers's "subliminal Self" is the name he gives, not to a second personality distinct from the primary personality and from time to time invading it, but to that larger portion of the whole personality which is experimentally known only when it succeeds in crossing the threshold which separates the subliminal from the supraliminal self. But this in some ways quite valuable conception does not tell us whether the subliminal Self is what it is by virtue of its past experiences, or by virtue of revelations made *in* it by a power which is not itself so much as an overshadowing Spirit seeking to draw the supraliminal Self into union. That is to say, we are not told by the doctrine of the "subliminal Self" whether what comes from it is but the result of the stimulation into intense activity of neural and psychical dispositions or complexes which were waiting for the clock to strike, or whether it is the result of a communication from what we have called the "transcendental Subject." The difference is the difference between exclusive mechanism and mechanism joined to self-determination. In the first case Spiritual Healing is the result of touching the button from outside which sets the machinery going, and in the second it is spiritual in the strict sense of being the free act of a self-determining being who finds himself *in* a mechanical complex and knows how to use it. It is to the former of these two conceptions to which it would seem desirable to limit the term sub-conscious; it then is a convenient term for each person's own protoplasm as differentiated by its age-long germinal life of action and reaction. The mind as well as the body is an instrument which does not lend itself to caprice or non-causality, but is, on the contrary, mechanically determined and so mechanically intelligible. The recognition of this indisputable fact is a preliminary step to the understanding of Spiritual Healing.

Spiritual Healing and Dreams.—The fact that both in pre-Christian and in Christian times dreams were largely used as a means of securing not only knowledge of how to get Spiritual Healing, but of getting it actually through the dream, led us to consider next the relation of dreams to Spiritual Healing. And we began, as was natural, with a description of the teaching of one of the best-known living authorities on the subject, Dr. Freud of Vienna. But Dr. Freud is mainly concerned with the dreams which may be regarded as the uneasy stirrings of the sub-conscious Self (as just defined), and to be explained, therefore, by the application of the Law of Causality. The mode of explanation consists in the dragging from their lair all the hidden delusions which serve to cause the wheels of the psychic chariot to go heavily, and in so applying the oil of rationality which is supplied by consciousness that all now goes smoothly. This enables the Life of the (to us) Unconscious to flow through our mind and body, and wash away all obstacles in either to its free and harmonious activities. And thus Dr. Freud's method would seem to be not so much a kind of Spiritual Healing as a useful discipline by which Spiritual Healing in the true sense becomes possible.

But it seems impossible to evade the force of the evidence both from ancient and modern times, which goes to show that under the head of dreams are many which are something more than mental constructions taking their starting-point in some event of the day before the night when the dream occurs—something more, even, than what Hippocrates meant when he said that "in dreams the soul knows the causes of disease, at least in an image." We refer to dreams such as the famous dream of Canon Warburton of Winchester, a man, as all who knew him would testify, of unimpeachable integrity and cool judgment. It is worth quoting here, as an example of this sort is better than all theorizing.[1]

"THE CLOSE, WINCHESTER,
"*July* 16, 1883.

"Somewhere about the year 1848 I went up from Oxford to stay a day or two with my brother, Acton Warburton, then a barrister, living at 10, Fish Street, Lincoln's Inn. When I got to his chambers I found a note on the table apologizing for his absence, and saying that he had gone to a dance somewhere in the West End, and intended to be at home soon after one o'clock. Instead of going to bed, I dozed in an arm-chair, but started up wide

[1] It is given in *Phantasms of the Living*, i. 338.

awake exactly at one, ejaculating, ' By Jove, he's
down ! ' and seeing him coming out of a drawing-
room into a brightly illuminated landing, catching
his foot in the edge of the top-stair, and falling
headlong, just saving himself by his elbows and
hands. (The house was one which I had never
seen, nor did I know where it was.) Thinking very
little of the matter, I fell a-doze again for half-an-
hour, and was awakened by my brother suddenly
coming in and saying, ' Oh, there you are ! I
have just had as narrow an escape of breaking my
neck as I ever had in my life. Coming out of the
ball-room, I caught my foot and tumbled full length
down the stairs.'
"That is all. It may have been ' only a dream,'
but I always thought it must have been ' something
more.' "

In that "something more" resided and still
resides the explanation of Spiritual Healing.
Spiritual Healing and Suggestion.—From the
psychical analysis of the Freudian School we then
passed to the Suggestion which is the last word of
explanation given at this moment by medical
science. And this led us naturally to one pronounced form of Suggestion, that known as Hypnotism. Hypnotism is the term by which Dr. Braid
covered his passage from the objective to the subjective, and substituted the phenomena of artificially
induced sleep for those of prânic energy. It by no
means follows, however, that because Hypnotism
discloses one well-marked series of facts, "mesmerism " is therefore discredited. Both may be

modes of reality, each occupying a lawful place in the scheme of things, and both capable of being used in the work of Spiritual Healing. A difference, however, of reputation now attaches to them. Hypnotism has received the imprimatur at last of the medical authority, while Prânism is still officially unrecognized. Yet anybody who cares to take even a very little trouble may easily satisfy himself that "magnetic healers," who are by no means scarce, do actually heal by virtue of the radiating force which we have suggested above should be called Prâna.

After noting Dr. Milne Bramwell's able discussion of hypnotic theories and the reference to Suggestion in Sir Douglas Powell's Note to the "Report of the Clerical and Medical Committee," we proceeded to inquire whether that Committee or the medical world in general has sufficiently considered the fact that Suggestion is, after all, little more than a name for the smallest part of the mysterious process of which it is made to cover the whole.

Mass-Suggestion.—Mass-suggestion is the name given to that collective and all-pervading psychical force which governs the minds of the members of a crowd, or of individuals subjected to the mood of a crowd. And the first example we took of this suggestion (which is all the more powerful because unconscious) was that afforded by Lourdes. The Roman Catholic writers who are in the habit of denying that Suggestion plays any part at Lourdes at all, forget for the most part the powerful stimuli set in activity by all the circumstances of the place. What is true of the Mass-suggestion exercised at Lourdes is also true of Treves, of St. Anne de Beaupré, of Loretto with its 50,000 pilgrims annually, of La Salette with 60,000, the "leaping procession" of Echternach with 25,000, the sanctuaries of Aix-le-Chapelle with 60,000, and the "Holy Mount" at Görz. The appetite for wonders grows by what it feeds on, and the effect of Mass-suggestion may as readily fall on the side of non-beneficial "ecstasy" as on that which is the scene of "miraculous" cures. Of this fact the convulsionaries of St. Médard are a standing witness, or the running amok of the Malays, or the phenomena of Tarantism. They all serve to show that strong mass-suggestions can set going such powerful auto-suggestion that Spiritual Healing ensues if the suggestion makes for that direction.

Some Conclusions.—Then we came to what seemed some justifiable conclusions on the whole matter. The first was that the similarity of stories of Spiritual Healing in all ages, countries and religions afforded a strong presumption that we were face to face with a phenomenon which sprang from reality and not hallucination. From Epidauros to Christian Science is a far cry, but the whole road between the two is marked with inscriptions recording in almost identical language similar experiences of Spiritual Healing. Can we escape from the inference that this undesigned coincidence between cures so widely different in place and time is due, not to accident, but to the fact that a constant force is at work doing the same thing in the same circumstances?

And if the results show a similarity, so, too, do the means employed. Something more than blind acceptance of tradition or superstitious trust in the outward observance of religious rites, surely must be invoked if we are to maintain a properly scientific attitude. We may well believe that Spiritual Healing is an actual fact because it springs from cosmic forces of a constant character. Among these we may, without fear of any taunt of obscurantism, include unseen spirits or personalities of some sort. The ancient belief in demons and angels has been looked at askance for some four centuries now in obedience to a one-sided rationalism, but there are signs of its revival, and our great anxiety may be not to get rid of it, but merely to apply the lesson which the history of superstition teaches so clearly, viz. that the belief in spirits requires careful watching and vigilant criticism if it is not to degenerate into pernicious sentimentalism, or fraud, or worse.

This led us to the subject of Faith. This is the name we give to the subjective factor which co-operates with the objective Force—whether this latter be mediated by personal beings or otherwise —in the work of Spiritual Healing. But when we call this Power God, we do not mean that God works on His world from outside it, but that He is Himself in some form or other the inner health-giving and organizing Principle which reaches from one end of the heaven to the other mightily, and sweetly ordereth all things. Whether this Principle work directly on the organism or work through finite centres on it, *i. e.* through personalities in the flesh or out of it, makes no difference. The result in Spiritual Healing is due to an inherent Power rearranging its materials, now exalting and now depressing them, creating no new thing, but changing what was, in order that what was not might become. Thus there is produced no "miracle" in the usual sense, but a result which is marvellous, is within Nature, and is the mark of a direct activity of God.

When this is stated in rational terms we are face to face with a truth which is the key to the phenomena of Spiritual Healing, the truth of the transcendental Self. Man is two Selves, one real and one illusory. The former is a member of the eternal, that is, the timeless order, and is embodied in a material organism. This organism creates the sense of the ordinary Ego of waking consciousness, whereas that Ego is but a pale reflection of the great overshadowing reality which is the transcendental Self. When the lower self can come into vital union with the higher Self, the road is cleared along which can travel the health-giving forces of the Great Physician. And their working it is which we detect in every marvel of Spiritual Healing. Moreover, that which links the lower self to the higher Self is that expectant, trusting, loving and receptive activity which in religion goes by the name of Faith. This great truth about the power of the transcendental Self and the illusory character of the lower self is what seems to be meant by Christian Science in the more or less unintelligible language of *Science and Health*. Hence the great importance of self-discipline, especially in the matter of the five great sources of disease, Fear, Anger, Lust, Envy and Jealousy. Finally, in this connection we were led to repeat that "Suggestion" says nothing and explains nothing, and suffers, too, from the bad philosophy which seems to underlie it as an explanation, viz. that something is transmitted from the suggester to his patient, as Force is vulgarly thought to be transmitted from the cueball to the object-ball in billiards.

This led us to the conclusion that Prayer at its highest and best is the expression of that Faith which constitutes the necessary subjective factor in Spiritual Healing. Nor is it to be thought that the case of Gabriel Gargam is any exception. Faith is not belief, and may co-exist with any sort of intellectual formulation of belief. A professed atheist may believe, as he says, in none of the religions he finds before him, and yet this negative attitude of his may have as its counterpart a hidden, inarticulate, and even unconscious devotion to the great central truth of all religion. The Healer and the patient may be bound in the same bundle of life by countless threads all too fine for our mortal eyes to see. The form that the healing process takes may be labelled as magnetic, mental, spiritualistic, or medical, but the process itself is not affected by these distinctions. They are merely convenient pigeon-holes for our thoughts about Spiritual Healing; Spiritual Healing itself is the same activity whether the "suggestion" is done by a pill or by a prayer. The Thinker is the physician, and this Thinker is divine.

Miracles.—Last of all, it did seem necessary to

orientate ourselves properly to a point of view which awakens confident asseveration and equally confident protestations. Roman Catholics assert "miracle" and are then silent as if they had thereby stated an explanation, whereas they have only started a battle-cry as *nichtssagend* as "suggestion." The quarrel, indeed, between those who look to the miraculous as the cause of Spiritual Healing and those who insist that whatever it may be it cannot be outside the realm of mechanical intelligibility is largely a question of words. The two are in a relation of what logicians call contrariety not of contradiction. Both in some sense may be true. And what the advocates of the miraculous seem concerned about is to make sure of the freedom of God to act as a Person on us as persons. What the scientific man defends with equal passion is the orderliness of the whole. He does not claim that we know all there is to know, but he is sure, a thousand times sure, that whatever else comes out of the unfathomed depths of Nature will not contradict anything already known and certified. It will modify but not destroy, and he looks askance, therefore, and rightly, at all assertions about the abrogation, violation or suspension of Nature's laws, for if these words mean what they say, then the world is no longer a cosmos, but has become once more *pro tanto* a chaos. And this is to undo all that science lives to do.

But the difficulty seems to disappear when we recognize that all change is of spiritual origin, that it is worked from within and not from without, and is all alike marvellous. The great miracle is not that some sick folk are instantaneously cured at a healing shrine, but that we all keep as well as we do under the operation of the constant and utterly trustworthy forces of a beneficent Nature. The making much of the exceptional in contradistinction to the ordinary is one sure sign of an undeveloped or perverted mind, or the substitution of a false religion for the true. It is anyhow clear that the earthly life of Jesus Christ was marked by works of Spiritual Healing, which seemed to come from Him as a matter of course when the occasion was favourable, and also that He distinctly and emphatically passed His condemnation on the spirit which trusted in signs and wonders. Where all the world is full of wonder, His personality is the greatest wonder of all. Its most wonderful manifestation was to be seen in His works of Spiritual Healing, and they were all as natural as they were wonderful. Spiritual Healing is a part of Nature's activity. Medical science, therefore, has no reason for denying it, but every reason for open-eyed investigation of it, and for applying it through its high-priests, whose training, we might be allowed to say in closing, would be the more efficient if provision were made in it for some better understanding of the transcendental as well as of the empirical side of man's complex being.

APPENDIX A

THE British Medical Council appointed in January 1909 a Sub-Committee to investigate and report on the whole question of Spiritual Healing, and care was taken to make it representative of the different branches of the profession by including on it general practitioners, physicians, neurologists and alienists. Its Report, printed in the *British Medical Journal*,[1] after describing in sections 1 to 7 the methods of its working, proceeds to give its general conclusions in sections numbered 8 to 16 as under—

8. The *modus operandi* adopted in "Spiritual Healing" consists in the laying on of hands and offering up of prayer by the "healer" in surroundings of a more or less impressive character.

9. After carefully considering the various definitions submitted to it, and the evidence afforded by its investigations, the Sub-Committee is of opinion that there is no difference in kind between "Spiritual Healing," "Faith Healing," "Mental Healing," and "Psychic Healing." All these forms seem to depend for their effect upon what is known as "Mental Suggestion."

10. No evidence has been brought before the Sub-Committee which would bear out the contention often urged by so-called "Spiritual Healers" that a special "Gift of Healing" is possessed by them.

11. Suggestion, as is well known, exercises a powerful effect in some cases of disease, principally those designated "functional," and the Sub-Committee believes it to be the essential factor in the cures wrought by means variously designated as above.

[1] Supplement, July 15, 1911, p. 125 ff.

12. Curative suggestion may be brought into operation by various means, such as the personal influence of one person over another, reinforced by appropriate surroundings as in the consulting-room of the physician; by excitement engendered under the influence of the claims made publicly by the quack, as seen frequently in the cures wrought on public platforms; by the atmosphere of ecstasy and expectation pervading a shrine such as "Lourdes"; and there is no reason to doubt that it may be induced by prayer and the laying-on of hands by the "Spiritual Healer" or by the priest. The surroundings may be different; the agent appears to be the same. In each case the receptive mental attitude of the patient is a most important factor.

13. The investigations of the Sub-Committee have satisfied it that the ministrations of the "Spiritual Healer," as of any other person skilfully using suggestion in its various forms, may cure functional disorders and alleviate pain in organic disease. No evidence has been forthcoming of any authenticated cure of organic disease. The undoubted subjective improvement noted in some cases of organic disease treated by "Spiritual Healing" can be equally obtained by treatment by other forms of suggestion for which no spiritual or supernatural claims are made. It seems to be mainly due to the spirit of hope and cheerfulness with which the patients are inspired, and which is often noted in similar cases at the beginning of a course of treatment hitherto untried. So far as such improvement, temporary though it be, occurs in cases of organic disease, the method of treatment must be credited with it. There is, however, grave danger that this subjective improvement may buoy the patient up with false hopes, and may induce him to refrain from seeking proper treatment until it is too late.

14. The Sub-Committee is confirmed in the opinion that the diagnosis and treatment of disease should be confined to those who have been trained with that end in view. Occasional cases of alleviation, or even apparent cure, of disease are not a sufficient set-off to

the risks which must be run when unqualified persons meddle with things which they cannot, from want of the appropriate training, understand.

15. So far as the ministrations of a priest may be helpful, as they undoubtedly are, in certain cases of illness, the medical man, whose business it is to cure his patient by any means at his disposal, will naturally and gladly avail himself of them.

16. The Sub-Committee is of opinion that the co-operation at present existing between the medical profession and the clergy in cases of sickness is often helpful to all concerned. Such co-operation has hitherto been of an informal nature, and has been governed by the circumstances of each case as it arose. The Sub-Committee can see no advantage in any more formal alliance, such as has, for example, been instituted in the United States, where clinics have been established in which certain cases, after being diagnosed by medical practitioners, are handed over to clergymen for treatment. Such a formal partnership, it is believed, is certain to set up in the minds, both of the clergy and of the public, erroneous ideas as to the nature of the education and qualifications necessary for the proper treatment of disease. The use of suggestion is within the power of all medical men to a greater or less degree, and when the practitioner feels that he would like further assistance, he can obtain it from physicians who are specially skilled in this department of medicine. Where the kind of suggestion that is set up by religious influence is specially needed, the practitioner will no doubt be able to secure the assistance of the clergyman or other person whose influence over the patient is likely to be most effective.

APPENDIX B

Report of Clerical and Medical Committee of Inquiry into Spiritual, Faith, and Mental Healing.[1]

The Committee fully recognize that the operation of the Divine Power can be limited only by the Divine Will, and desire to express their belief in the efficacy of prayer.

They reverently believe, however, that the Divine Power is exercised in conformity with, and through the operation of, natural laws. . . .

The Committee are of opinion that the physical results of what is called "Faith" or "Spiritual" Healing do not prove on investigation to be different from those of Mental healing or healing by "Suggestion." The term Suggestion is used in this Report in a wide sense, as meaning the application of any natural mental process to the purposes of treatment.

They recognize that Suggestion is more effectively exercised by some persons than by others, and this fact seems to explain the "gifts" of a special character claimed by various "Healers." . . .

They are aware that no sharply defined fundamental distinction can be drawn between "organic" and "functional" ailments. They are forced, however, to the conclusion, after the most careful inquiry, that "Faith" or "Spiritual" healing, like all treatment by suggestion, can be expected to be permanently effective only in cases of what are generally termed "functional" disorders. The alleged exceptions are so disputable that they cannot be taken into account. . . .

While making this statement they thankfully recognize that persons suffering from organic disease are greatly comforted and relieved, and even physically

[1] This Report is abbreviated here, as much of it is of a desultory character. What is quoted is all that is definite in the Conclusions of the Report. It was issued in the spring of 1914.

benefited by spiritual ministrations. Such ministrations, by appealing to the spiritual nature and reinforcing the spiritual powers, may contribute greatly to the success of the physical treatment by the medical practitioner.

APPENDIX C [1]

I

We give in this Appendix the Creed of Mesmer, the two professional Reports made on it, and the Minority Report of de Jussieu.

The Twenty-seven Articles of the Creed of Mesmer.

1. There is a natural influence exerted on each other by the heavenly bodies, the earth and animated bodies.

2. The means of this influence is a fluid universally dispersed and continuous, admitting of no vacuum, the subtlety of which is beyond all comparison, which by its nature is capable of receiving, propagating, and communicating all forms of motion.

3. This reciprocal action is governed by mechanical laws which at present are unknown.

4. There results from this action rhythmic movements which may be regarded as ebb and flow.

5. This ebb and flow is more or less general, more or less special, more or less complex according to the causes which govern it.

6. It is by this activity (the most general of all revealed in Nature) that active relations subsist between the heavenly bodies, the earth, and its constituent members.

7. On this activity depend the properties of matter and organisms.

The documents given in this Appendix are translated from C. Burdin and Fred Dubois, *Histoire Académique du magnétisme animal*, Paris, chez T. B. Baillière, 1841.

U

8. The animal body experiences the rhythmic movements of this agent, which insinuates itself into the nervous system and so affects it immediately.

9. There are manifested, particularly in the human body, properties analogous to those of the magnet; in both are poles different and opposed which can be communicated, changed, destroyed and reinforced. Even the phenomenon of inclination is observed in it.

10. Seeing that the property of the animal body, which makes it susceptible of the influence of the heavenly bodies and of the reciprocal action of those which surround it, is analogous to the property of the magnet, I have been led to call it *animal magnetism*.

11. The active force of animal magnetism so characterized can be communicated to other bodies animate and inanimate; these are, however, susceptible in different degrees.

12. This active force can be reinforced and propagated by these same bodies.

13. Experience shows the passage of a matter whose subtlety penetrates all bodies, without undergoing any appreciable loss.

14. Its action takes place at a distance without the help of any intermediate body.

15. It is increased and reflected by glasses like the former.[1]

16. It is communicated, propagated and increased by sound.

17. This magnetic force can be accumulated, concentrated and transported.

18. I have said that animate bodies are not equally susceptible of this force; there are some even, though rarely found, which have so opposite a property that their presence alone destroys all the effects of this magnetism in other bodies.

19. This opposite power in its turn penetrates all bodies; it, too, can be communicated, propagated, accumulated, concentrated, transported, reflected by glasses, and propagated by sound; this makes it to be not a mere privation but a positively opposite force.

[1] Magnetism.

20. The magnet, whether natural or artificial, is, like all other bodies, susceptible of animal magnetism, and even of the opposite force, without in either case its action on iron and the needle suffering any alteration; this proves that the principle of animal magnetism differs essentially from that of mineral magnetism.

21. This system will throw fresh light on the nature of fire and light, as well as on the theory of attraction, of the positive and negative aspects of magnetism and electricity.

22. It must be recognized that magnetism and electricity, artificially induced, have in relation to illness only properties common to several other agents in Nature, and that when there have resulted from their application any beneficial effects, these are due to animal magnetism.

23. It will be seen from the facts arising out of the practical rules which I shall lay down that this principle can cure immediately nerve troubles and others mediately.

24. With its help the doctor is enlightened as to the use of drugs whose action it perfects; moreover it provokes and directs salutary crises so as to assume the mastery over them.

25. In communicating my method, I shall show by a new theory of diseases the universal utility of the principle with which I combat them.

26. With this knowledge the doctor will diagnose accurately the origin, the nature, and the progress of diseases, even the most complicated; he will prevent their getting worse, and will succeed in curing them without at any time exposing the patient to danger of lapse, whatever his age, temperament or sex; women in a state of pregnancy and apart from child-birth will enjoy the same advantage.

27. This doctrine, in short, will put the doctor in a position to judge of the degree of health of each individual, and to preserve him from the illnesses to which he may be exposed; the art of healing will thus arrive at its final perfection.

II

Report of the Committee appointed by King Louis XVI of France to inquire into Animal Magnetism.

The King nominated, March 12, 1784, from the Medical Faculty of Paris, MM. Borrie, Sallin, d'Arcet, and Guillotin, and at the request of these four men he added, from the Royal Academy of Sciences, MM. Franklin, le Roy, Bailly, de Bouy, and Lavoisier. The Report was signed by the nine members (except that Majault took the place of Borrie) on August 11, 1784. The conclusion only is reproduced here.

"The Commissioners, having recognized that this animal-magnetic fluid can be perceived by none of our senses, that it has had no effect whether on themselves or on the sick on whom they have experimented; being assured that pressures and touches cause changes which are seldom favourable to the animal economy, and also violent agitations in the imagination which are always pernicious; having finally proved by decisive experiments that imagination without magnetism produces convulsions, and that magnetism without imagination produces nothing :

"They have come to the conclusion unanimously, on the question of the existence and utility of magnetism, that there is no proof of the existence of animal-magnetic fluid, and that therefore there is no use in a fluid which has no existence; that the violent effects observed in treatment in public are due to touching, to the imagination set in action, and to that mechanical imitation which makes us, in spite of ourselves, repeat what strikes our senses.

"At the same time they feel themselves compelled to add, as an important remark, that the touchings, the repeated act of the imagination to produce the crises, can be injurious; that the sight of those crises is equally dangerous owing to that imitative power which seems to be a law of Nature; and that in consequence all public treatment where the means of magnetism are employed can only have, in the long run, disastrous consequences."

III

Report of the Committee of the Royal Society of Medicine named by the King to examine into Animal Magnetism.

This Committee was contemporaneous with the former, and issued its report August 16, 1784, which was signed by Poissonnier, Caille, Mauduyt and Audry. As before, the conclusions alone are quoted here.

Conclusions on the first part of our Report—the facts.

"1. There do not exist, even on the admission of M. Deslon,[1] any physical proofs of the existence of the agent or fluid which has been supposed to be the principle of *animal magnetism;*

"2. The proofs cited to prove the existence of this principle, drawn from internal sensations, are ambiguous, often illusory, and therefore always insufficient;

"3. The effects attributed to this unknown principle, which are regarded as proofs of its existence, depend on evident and known causes, from which it follows that the existence of the unknown agent or fluid, which is regarded as the principle of *animal magnetism,* is but an hypothesis void of support;

"4. What is called *animal magnetism,* reduced to its proper proportions by the examination and analysis of facts and circumstances, is only the art of preparing predisposed sensitive subjects, by accidental and concomitant circumstances already evaluated in this Report, for certain convulsive movements, and for exciting movements in those subjects by a determinate and immediate cause, without having recourse to the new agent whose existence has been postulated without any ground for it."

[1] A doctor and pupil of Mesmer.

Conclusions on the second part of our Report—the utility of the facts.

"It follows from the first part of our Report—

"1. That the pretended animal magnetism, such as it has been proclaimed in our day, is an ancient system, puffed in the preceding century and fallen into oblivion;

"2. That the advocates of animal magnetism, whether those who have put forward this system, or those who have resuscitated it among us, have never formerly, and cannot to-day, furnish any proof of the existence of the unknown agent or of the fluid to which they have attributed certain properties and certain workings, and that consequently the existence of such an agent is a gratuitous supposition;

"3. That what has been called *animal magnetism*, when reduced to its proper value after the examination and analysis of facts, is the art of causing sensitive people to fall into convulsions by touches applied to the most sensitive parts of the body, and by friction applied to those parts, after having predisposed those persons for such effects by numerous accompanying circumstances which can be varied at will, several of which are by themselves capable of provoking the strongest convulsions in certain cases and in certain subjects.

"4. We began the second part of our Report with the remark that if the pretended *animal magnetism*, famous in the last century, had been really useful, custom would have fixed and perpetuated it.

"5. We have made it clear that it is a mistake in the use of terms to talk of *coction* and *crises* as names for the effects produced by *animal magnetism;* that between the *coction* and the *crises,* which are the means which nature employs to heal, and the effects of pretended magnetism, there is no other relation than that of similarity of words, while all the essential and constituent conditions are diametrically opposite.

"6. We have set out in detail the many grave dangers to which people are exposed by the use of the pretended *animal magnetism;* we have insisted on the evils to be feared from the convulsions it excites and the evacuations of which it is the occasion.

"We therefore think—

"1. That the theory of *animal magnetism* is a system wholly devoid of proof;

"2. That this pretended means of healing, reduced to the irritation of sensitive parts, to imitation and the effects of imagination, is at least useless for those in whom there ensue no evacuations or convulsions, and that it may often become dangerous by provoking and over-stimulating the nervous system of hypersensitive persons;

"3. That it is injurious to those in whom it produces the effects improperly termed *crises;* that it is the more dangerous in proportion as the *crises* are more vehement, or the convulsions more violent, or the evacuations more thorough, and that in very many cases the consequences may be fatal;

"4. That the treatments performed in public in the display of *animal magnetism* unite to all the ills indicated above that besides of exposing a number of well-constituted persons to contract a spasmodic and convulsive disposition which may be the source of great evils;

"5. That these conclusions are to be taken to cover all that is offered to the public at the present time under the name of *animal magnetism,* since its machinery and its consequences being everywhere the same, the inconveniences and the dangers it arouses deserve everywhere the same treatment."

IV

De Jussieu's Report

As is well known, one of the Commissioners, Jussieu, presented a Minority Report, apparently because he thought the Report of the Majority too negative in its conclusions, as it was certainly illogical in its assertion that *animal magnetism* did not exist and yet might well be the cause of terrible evils. As Jussieu's position has often been misrepresented it may be worth while to quote so much from his Report as will make his position clear. He starts with asserting matter and motion as the two principles of living bodies, the latter being the immediate agent, under unalterable laws, of all animal functions. This force, "seeking always to establish an equilibrium, insinuates itself into some bodies and escapes from others by virtue of the quantity of it contained in each." It may be identified with the "electric principle which is dispersed in all bodies and exercises a similar sensible action." This force, which is ubiquitous, is in animated beings, such as plants and animals, the vital force, and as such obeys the same law of equilibrium, so that "every living being is a very veritable electrified body constantly filled with this active principle, but not always in the same proportion. It varies in different living beings and in different organs in the same individual." Each living being, therefore, is a radiating centre of this vital force, and this force will flow to one with a lower potential, or take in from another with a higher potential, or remain constant in presence of one with the same potential.

But in the higher animals there exists a higher principle from which proceed will and imagination, and these unlike physical causes are "special, inconstant and variable with each individual." We shall be chary, therefore, says Jussieu, of confusing "the action of soul and of imagination with the action that is merely animal," and will distinguish between the cause which determines and the agent which executes." And he thinks it would be easy to extend the comparison between the electric fluid and the active animal principle to prove more and more their identity. Finally, he maintains that what is being questioned may well be regarded as "animal heat," but "whatever it may be there anyhow exists a force which is neither will nor imagination; which exercises on bodies an uninterrupted activity; which exercises functions of all sorts, some without concurrence or help, some under the immediate direction of will and imagination; which receives also the direct influence of external physical causes; which, in a word, is always an intermediary agent, charged with the direct carrying-out of all movements that take place in man. . . . Heat, ever active, is then this real part which emanates from the body, that unknown and debated agent which constitutes the physical influence of man on man." His formal conclusion is as follows—

"The theory of magnetism can only be admitted when developed and backed by solid proof. The experiments performed to prove the existence of the magnetic fluid prove only that man exerts on his fellow a sensible action by friction, by contact, and less frequently by a mere proximity at some distance off. This effect attributed to a non-proven universal fluid, is due certainly to the animal heat existing in bodies, which constantly emanates from them, travels far, and can pass from one body to another. Animal heat is developed, increased or diminished in a body both by moral and physical causes. Judged by its effects, it is of the nature of tonic remedies, producing like them consequences advantageous or disadvantageous, according to the quantity and mode of its impartation. A more extended and more closely studied use of this agent will enable us better to understand its precise mode of acting and its utility."

These words go to show how much more in common there was between Jussieu's philosophy and Mesmer's beliefs than between the conclusions of Jussieu and those of his colleagues, and make it difficult to understand how MM. Burdin and Dubois can say that "De Jussieu dans son interpretation est plus exclusif que ses collègues mais il n'est pas en contradiction avec eux."

APPENDIX D

APPENDIX D

STATEMENT BY BROTHER RAMANANDA

I WILL put into everyday words an account of some cases. My name can be used in any way you wish, for I am more glad than I can say to be able to help you to awaken in human nature the knowledge of the real meaning of *Spirit* and its *All Power*.

First I would like to draw attention to some cures of animals.

The first experience I can remember of healing is that as a wee child, whilst living with the "Holy Men," I used to live in such a "real" way, that neither the snows nor extreme heat had any effect on me.

I was in such harmony with God, as expressed through His earth and its occupants, that I was in no sense conscious of a contrast with anything. I could go and live with the wild animals. I was often in touch with large tigers, and have played and romped with their clubs. I was always alone physically in my rambles, only at certain hours of the day was I in association with my masters.

During my walks I was always in touch with other people with finer bodies than ordinary, for at that time mine was also in finer vibrations, and I was therefore in poise with those around. I have walked on water and glided through great ravines in the Himalayas. Near our summer residence, which was a forest, there was a pool of water where each season storks used to come to breed, and they would always ask me to come at the time of hatching.

I remember, though only four or five years of age, gliding on the water to their nest, over which they were standing in the water, as is their custom. Sometimes I would wade out as I grew older. I have handled many, so called, dangerous snakes and have been carried by panthers.

To come to the points of healing God's smaller creatures : Frogs, on the above-mentioned water, would sometimes be attacked by hawks, and, though I was only two or three, I well remember my first experience of healing was the replacing of the flesh and skin on these frogs' backs which had been torn by the hawks dropping them on my approach. I would caress the frogs for a while, and always saw a fine white doughy substance envelop them, and I would watch the wounded flesh quickly mend and the skin be replaced, and lastly the green colour and brown markings reappear as they were originally.

One day a big tiger met me near a water-hole with a very inflamed paw. A large splinter was in it. As he came up to me I saw this same substance enveloping him.

Now this is a point to which I wish to draw attention to show that it was not my power that healed at that time. I was about twelve years of age and in a much less *real* state, for my father had formed a desire for me to devote myself to modern Western life, instead of spending the years until I was twenty-five in developing the Spiritual. These cross vibrations would have tended to decrease any power I personally had had, so, as this dear beast had desired healing, it was then reaching him. Whether my practical help was needed for complete realization I cannot say. The same law applies in this case as in that of human beings. Where two or three are together in His Name the Living Life manifests.

I took his paw in my hand before turning it over—he had then lain down at my feet—a large piece of black wood came out and fell at my feet, and almost instantly I saw the tendons move into place, the flesh knit together, skin grow over and new hair come through, this wonderful substance moving in cloud-like waves all the time. Sometimes in spiral waves with great rapidity, a wonderful golden light was directed into the region of his solar plexus. After a few minutes of such working, he jumped up and leaped right over me, crouching down and licking my feet, hands and face.

Many such instances I can quote. Other cases of

animals, birds, etc., were treated with manipulations, and some were of slower healing. Once in Australia I came across a large iguana, four feet long, like a small crocodile, that had been caught in a spring trap. He was scratching and squirming, and had dug up the earth in his agony. His paw, as big as a boy's hand, was nearly cut off. He allowed me to unspring the trap and lift the paw out. Only gnawed sinews were holding it together, he had tried to chew it off in his desire to free himself.

He crawled over my knees and held his head up, and the same beautiful light appeared and was directed to him; the broken limb mended instantly, he turned and faced me and crouched down, and for ten minutes we remained in silence as the sun went down, then he turned slowly away and crawled up a gum-tree whole and happy.

Innumerable cats, fowls, dogs, horses and cattle I have seen healed in the same way. Many times sheep which were half-picked to death by crows whilst lambing were healed. More recently several horses were brought to me in Jersey, one with fearful broken wind was healed at once. An Aberdeen terrier with a fearful patch of mange on his back would often come up to us on the beach and look so mournful. I am sorry to say that, for a week, we always drove him away. One day a linking up with him came over me, and I called him, much to his delight, and I concentrated for a while for his relief. Next day hair had begun to grow, and in a week he was well.

So in such cases of healing animals, which I feel to be just as important as humans, I feel it is no peculiar power bestowed on me, for I am an outside witness of the psychological moment when (creatures and humans) they realized the greatness of Spirit beside the delusion of material unpoise. The kind of co-operation employed does not matter. The special time comes when they seek, the door is opened and entry can be had, completely or otherwise. Maybe the means co-operated with acts as oil to the door, or even turned the handle, but the power to realize it is within the individual himself. I have seen instantaneous realizations in individuals of—outwardly judging—low spiritual growth, and in cases of advanced souls, long periods occur before they make the slightest headway in the physical expression of the awakening life within.

(1) Six or seven years ago, whilst in Chicago, I had a case of a boy whose arm had been completely crushed from the wrist to the elbow by a motor-car, the bones were splintered and protruding through the flesh; pieces of gravel and asphalt were embedded in it. A medical man whom I had employed at my place suggested amputation. The boy was unconscious—no possibility of taking suggestion verbally; I saw a great power working within him, and as I was praying I felt healing was taking place. In less than five minutes his arm was perfect, not even a trace of blood could be seen.

(2) A Colonel of U.S.A. army had the forefinger of the left hand bent. He was born, as the doctors said, with no middle joint, but with one solid bone. One day I was motoring with my mother, and he passed in his car. Seeing me, he stopped behind my car, and said : "I want this healed, so help me God." I said : "Yes, it is done now in His Name." He put out his hand, and the finger was straight. I did not touch him. As he called on God, I saw the finger loosening. No physical help from me came at all; the co-operation of Faith secured the result.

(3) A case of boy of fourteen, kicked in the back by horse. Kidneys misplaced, complete paralysis, for fifteen months, of legs from hips downwards—the lower organs not working, continual pain and abscesses. Made arrangements for operation. Kill or cure prospects. Two days before heard of me through girl who had been cured by distant treatment. First treatment boy walked, though his legs were like jelly. I laid on hands and told him to exercise legs as much as possible now that the life had come back to them. In ten days' time they were big and strong as if nothing had ever been the matter with them. This was four years ago. He writes to me weekly. He is now learn-

ing electrical engineering. Many people in Brisbane know of this case, and the doctors were amazed.

(4) A child of two-and-a-half years of age dying of tuberculosis of the bowels. Doctor said only half-an-hour to live; just skin and bone; smelt like a partially decomposed corpse. When treated, opened his eyes and began crying loudly, and would not stop until warm milk and biscuits were given him. Next day he was up on his feet after a long night's sleep. It was beautiful to see the blood rushing to his limbs. Where it came from no material laws can explain. To-day he is a chubby lad and growing tall. This was in a mining town in Australia.

I had in the same town several cases of miners' phthisis caused by bits of quartz getting into the lungs when the men are chipping the rock for gold. The big drilling-machines now used also cause many deaths from the lungs becoming riddled with splinters and dust of the quartz. The men suffer acutely. There is supposed to be no earthly cure. To prolong life the miners leave the work, but suffer always.

(5) The wife of a dean of the Church of England came to Australia for health. On the voyage inflammation of the ear came on, and it was so bad that an operation was attempted, though the boat was bad and the weather severe. The drum was completely ruined, and when they came to me it was destroyed. My mother and I knelt in silent prayer. She opened her eyes, and, gazing at some beautiful vision, remained as if listening for ten minutes, and then said she could hear perfectly. The other ear had been partly deaf also.

A manager of a big drapery establishment had a similar experience. He had been born with only one ear-drum, and the inability to hear in his work was very trying. In his case the doctors laughed, until they examined the ear and there saw complete new workings.

(6) A lady had been given up by four doctors after a consultation. They said her only chance was to have a leg amputated as mortification had set in, owing to some fearful complication of the spleen, which in some

way had affected the big blood-vessels of the leg. The leg was horrible to look at. That night my mother and I were called in to treat her, although she was under the influence of a narcotic. She had many friends in the house, and they all gathered round her bed. My mother prayed that we should realize the great awakening in each one of us, and after I laid on hands, she opened her eyes and got up. Next day all inflammation had gone. The leg and the internal disorder were quite well in a week. To-day she is touring in the mountains of New Zealand, though over seventy years of age. This was over four years ago.

(7) Case of woman who, eighteen years ago, was trodden on by a horse. She had gone to the horse's head, when the horse reared up and planted his forefeet in the small of her back. The doctors said that her back was broken and there was no hope, but she held to the "dear Healing of Jesus," as she expressed it, and she lived on for fifteen years with the help of plaster of Paris coats, etc., and, though in great pain and always on her back, she trusted that one day she would be whole.

I was visiting the clergyman of her church in the State of Victoria, Australia. She had told him about that time that Christ was coming to heal her through one of His workers—not even the minister knew of my work at that time. One day, after a service in one of his churches, we went to this woman's house for a midday meal. As I stepped into the doorway, though she could not see me, she said : "The Beloved had, at last, sent a messenger." We prayed, and she was at once made whole, and now is daily bringing many to the knowledge of their at-one-ment with God.

(8) I have seen many cases healed before reaching me whilst treating after services. They would start hobbling along on crutches and sticks or being led, but so eager were they to be whole, that the self-healing expressed itself as they sought my co-operation. One case of a man with tuberculosis of the hip, the right side drawn down, right leg shorter than the other, pieces of bone working through, was healed

before reaching the platform. Next day he called on me, walking straight and with the legs of equal length.

Many cures are only very gradual. I have had many children with withered limbs cured at once, and many, of course, of slower growth, in which cases, massage, etc., causes the filling out.

When once the vital current has been started, if we help in natural and practical ways, God will help us.

(9) A curate was cured instantly of cataract. He was nearly blind. The growth peeled off like a skin from fruit. At his church I went to Communion with an old woman of eighty-four, with bad inflamed eyes—a kind of catarrh. We had arranged that she would realize the Bread and Wine as the Living Life and I would feel likewise. When she got up from the Altar rail, the light from the windows was so strong (both natural and spiritual light) she was amazed, and was becoming somewhat excited, but a great calmness came over her, and on regaining our seats, she remained in prayer for twenty minutes. I believe to this day her eyes are bright and clear.

(10) A Chinaman, with cancer in the tongue, who had been refused treatment by Western doctors, by reason of the Australian dislike of the yellow race, and the then considered uselessness of operation for cancer, was healed at once; it is true that I cut off a growth under the tongue, but I need not have done so, for when we prayed, the cure was so complete that no mark was shown, and even the part I had taken out, though placed in a dish with water and wadding, had disappeared, leaving clear water and clean wadding. This shows the returning to its proper vibration of that which has been in touch with Reality.

(11) Man with erysipelas of leg, very bad, had been getting worse and worse for seventeen years, cured completely in three weeks.

(12) Boy in London having finger cut off except skin on one side; sewed on bone; would not knit; amputation decided on, boy believing it would get better without it. I was at the doctor's house. The doctor

showed me the finger, and said could anything be done to it, other than operation? The doctor desired me to treat him, and he himself concentrated too. Result: next day the doctor wrote to say bone knit perfectly well. Three weeks after saw lad, and the finger was well.

(13) Distant case of sclerosis in Ireland. Letter to say that it was quite cured after three weeks of daily meditation on his part, feeling whilst so doing that the Indweller was at work.

Here I will say that in my helping of distant cases I do not concentrate specially for individuals at various times of the day, but I always meditate from two to five a.m.; then I enter into the state of illumination and so centre the "White Light," that all those who desire healing at various times of the day can tap this great store and thereby utilize it. In this way I eliminate the possibility of my thought-life and that of my daily environment coming into contact with the patients. Also it proves again that the results are due to self-healing. The letters to say that they felt my presence at such and such a time are innumerable, but, to me, stand for nothing, for I always put myself in harmony with the Universal and not the Particular.

(14) Case of doctor in England with Bright's disease and eruption over back and stomach, cured by following out my directions in meditation.

(15) Mother and child in Jersey, given up by six doctors—consumption. Mother ill for years; child three weeks old; the day we were called in, given up. As we prayed, a wonderful representation of the Holy Mother and Child appeared, and a great power was felt. Both became perfectly well. In Jersey the work was very good, dozens weekly regaining perfect health.

In India, where miracles are expected by all classes, wonderful things happen through that simple faith. I have had many cases of leprosy healed instantly. It was most weird to see the white kind getting well, to see big white patches on dark skin getting dark and regaining their natural colour. Jersey people exhibit direct faith, as in the East—not faith in human beings,

x

but in God. I have seen the most obstinate cases of neuritis made well, asthma, in some dozens of cases, cured, and flesh cut and broken through accidents healed at once.

(16) Two babies, three and four weeks old, cousins, were brought to me covered with disease, eyes unopened, faces one mass of sores; they became well in few days. Many cases of sterile men and women were, by the Inner Awakening, restored to their full functions. Cases of perverted menstruation were rectified. I knew very little of the cases at the time when the sufferers came to me, and I do not often know the seat of the disease at the time of healing. Nor do I always know the precise nature of the malady, but I believe, and know the All Pervading will do what He knows is required.

Healing, however performed, does not interfere with Karma, or in any way abrogate the Law of cause and effect, for the Christian Bible says that all men can be *saved*, and that word "saved" means to us in the East *liberation* from the unreal. Hence no matter what the cause may be, both cause and effect *can* be transcended at any time, if man will only look within, casting aside Mâyâ, and seek ever Mahsua (which is liberation from the bonds of matter), and the Glory of Him the Beloved One—God.

All works of healing bear testimony to God's power, which is ever ready to be used, be it individually or collectively, with or without the knowledge of the patient. It is not a matter of "putting into the head" of a patient this truth. Many cases where the individual is so confused that clear thinking is seemingly impossible *can* be cured by the knowledge that *Spirit is in all*.

BIBLIOGRAPHY

BERTRIN, GEORGES : *Histoire Critique des Événements de Lourdes*, 1912.

BOSANQUET, BERNARD : *The Principle of Individuality and Value*, 1912. Of quite exceptional importance.

BRAMWELL, J. MILNE : *Hypnotism, its History, Practice and The ry :* third edition, 1913, pp. 480. The most comprehensive work in English on the subject, and the one in which the rationale of the practice of hypnotism is most thoroughly dealt with.

BRINTON, DANIEL G. : *The Myths of the New World*, 1896.

BUCKLEY, J. M., LL.D. : *Faith-healing, Christian Science and Kindred Phenomena*, 1892, pp. 291. Discursive, but full of useful information ; critical.

BURDIN, C., and DUBOIS, FRED : *Histoire Académique du Magnetisme animale*, 1841. Sceptical.

COBB, I. GEIKIE, M.D. : Articles on "Neurasthenia," *Practitioner*, October 1912, April 1913, June 1914; *Medical World*, October 23, 1913, January 24, 1914.

DEUBNER, LUDWIG : *Kosmas und Damian*, Teubner, 1907.
         "   *De Incubatione*,   "   1900.

DIETERICH, ALBRECHT : *Abraxas*, Teubner, 1891.

DU PREL, CARL : *Philosophy of Mysticism*, trans. C. C. Massey, two vols., 1889. An admirable treatment of the *meaning* and psychology of the phenomena of Hypnotism ; should not be overlooked. It has no index.

ENQUIRER, AN : *A Plea for the thorough and unbiassed Investigation of Christian Science*, 1913.

FEILDING, ALICE : *Faith-healing and Christian Science*, 1899, pp. 214. Useful and sound.

FLAMMARION, CAMILLE : *L'Inconnu*, Eng. trans. (*The Unknown*), Harper, 1900.

GLIDDON, AURELIUS, J. L. : *Faith Cures, their History and Mystery*, 1896, pp. 211. A convenient summary.

HAMILTON, MARY : *Incubation*, 1906. The best English book on the subject.

HARNACK, ADOLF : *Medicinisches aus der Ältesten Kirchengeschichte*, Leipzig. 1892.
—— *Die Mission und Ausbreitung des Christentums*, 1902.

HARRIS, J. RENDEL : *The Dioscuri in the Christian Legends*, 1903.

JONES, W. H. S.: *Malaria and Greek History*, to which is added, *The History of Greek Therapeutics and the Malaria Theory*, in "Publications of the University of Manchester," in which it is No. VIII of the Historical Series, 1909, pp. 156.

KUTSCH, FERDINAND: *Attische Heilgötter und Heilheroen*, Giessen, 1913.

LOTZE, HERMANN: *Microcosmus*, Eng. trans. 2 vols., 1885. Invaluable.

McDOUGALL, WILLIAM: *Body and Mind*, 1911. An able defence of Animism.

MANN, CHARLES H.: *Psychiasis, Healing through the Soul*, Boston, 1900, pp. 158. A sane treatment of the subject by a Minister of the "New Church."

MILMINE, GEORGINE: *The Life of Mary Baker G. Eddy*, New York, 1909, pp. 495. A history both of Mrs. Eddy and of her movement, documented and illustrated.

MOLL, ALBERT: *Hypnotism:* in the "Contemporary Science Series," 1890, pp. 408. Contains a useful chapter on "Animal Magnetism."

MYERS, F. W. H.: *Human Personality*, two vols., 1903 (one volume ed., abridgment of former, pub. 1907).

PAGET, STEPHEN: *The Faith and Works of Christian Science*, 1909, pp. 278. Severely critical.

PODMORE, FRANK: *Mesmerism and Christian Science*, 1909.

POWELL, LYMAN P.: *Christian Science, the Faith and its Founder*, 1907, pp. 261. An able and fair examination from the pen of an Episcopalian clergyman in the United States.

ROHDE, ERWIN: *Psyche*, Freiburg i. B., 1894.

SAYCE, A. H.: *The Religions of Ancient Egypt and Babylonia*, 1902.

STOLL, DR. OTTO: *Suggestion und Hypnotismus in der Völkerspsychologie;* 2nd ed., 1904, pp. 738. An invaluable work for the student, and a mine of information; it is deficient, however, in its psychological analysis, and has an inadequate index.

TERTULLIAN, Q. SEPT FLORENT: *De animâ.* The best early Christian witness.

TUCKEY, C. LLOYD: *Treatment by Hypnotism and Suggestion*, fifth edition, 1907, pp. 418.

TUKE, DANIEL HACK: *Illustrations of the Influence of the Mind upon the Body.* Two vols., second ed., 1884. Invaluable to the student.

WEINREICH, OTTO: *Antike Heilungswunder*, Giessen, 1909.

INDEX

Lightning Source UK Ltd.
Milton Keynes UK
UKHW011312061221
395182UK00002B/726